Cholesterol Lowering Cookbooks

Superfoods and Dairy Free for a Low Cholesterol Diet

Kelly Marcil

Table of Contents

CHOLESTEROL LOWERING COOKBOOKS INTRODUCTION 1

SECTION 1: SUPERFOODS INTRODUCTION 6

SALMON.. 8
Sweet Coconut Crusted Salmon...9
Salmon Quiche..11
Quick and Easy Pan Fried Salmon..13
Tunisian Style Baked Salmon 14
Baked Salmon with Lemon and Dill 16
Salmon Ceviche 17
Salmon – Cream Cheese Dip 19

SPINACH 20
Spinach, Lentil and Bean Curry 21
Beef Stew with Spinach 23
Curried Spinach and Chickpeas 25
Wilted Spinach Salad with Goat Cheese and Cherries.......................27
Baked Spinach and Feta Pitas 28
Chicken Florentine...30
Fruit and Spinach Smoothie...32

QUINOA 33
Baked Quinoa Breakfast Cereal 34
Five Spice Quinoa...35
Quinoa Pilaf 36
Quinoa and Mushrooms 38
Broccoli and Quinoa Soup 40
Quinoa Salad with Cranberries and Cilantro................................42

BEANS AND LENTILS 44
Vegetarian Chili 46

Pasta Fagioli 48

Cuban Style Black Beans.. 50

Black Bean Hummus 52

Southwestern Breakfast Platter............................... 53

Lentil Soup 54

Baked Chicken and Lentils...................................... 56

APPLES **58**

Apple Soup 59

Brown Rice Salad with Fruit and Nuts 61

Braised Escarole 62

Apple Coleslaw... 63

Apple Chutney.. 64

Apple Turnovers.. 65

Apple Crisp.. 67

YOGURT **69**

Yogurt Pound Cake.. 70

Yogurt Rice.. 72

Beet and Yogurt Salad.. 74

Yogurt Chicken... 75

Yogurt Parfait with Blueberries................................ 77

Haydari 78

Eggplant and Yogurt Salad...................................... 79

Yogurt Salad Dressing.. 81

Spinach Dip with Yogurt... 82

Turkish-Style Zucchini Salad 83

SWEET POTATOES **84**

Sweet and Spicy Sweet Potatoes 85

Sweet Potato Soup... 86

Sweet Potato Rolls... 88

Oven Roasted Sweet Potatoes................................... 90

Sweet Potato Chili 91

Sweet Potato Pie 93

Spicy Roasted Sweet Potatoes 95

Sweet Potato Fries 96

KIWI FRUIT 97

Kiwi Salsa 98
Spinach Salad with Kiwi and Strawberries 99
Kiwi Sandwiches..100
Kiwi Strawberry Smoothies 101
Fruit Pizza 102

BLUEBERRIES.. 103

Blueberry Pie..104
Blueberry Granita...105
Blueberry Salsa 106
Blueberry Chicken 107
Blueberry Walnut Salad 109

DARK CHOCOLATE 110

Spicy Dark Chocolate Cookies 111
Dark Chocolate Truffles...114

OATS 116

Bannocks (Scottish Oat Cakes)...117

PUMPKIN.. 119

New England Style Pumpkin Bread....................................120
Oatmeal with Pumpkin...122
Pumpkin Pasta...123
Pumpkin Tacos or Tostadas 125

SUPERFOODS CONCLUSION 127

SECTION 2: DAIRY FREE DIET 128

BENEFITS OF DAIRY FREE - WHY PEOPLE CHOOSE DAIRY FREE.. 130

HOW TO COPE WHEN YOU'RE A DAIRY LOVER, BUT

FOR HEALTH REASONS YOU MUST GO DAIRY FREE 133

SAMPLE 5 DAY DAIRY FREE DIET PLAN.....................137

KIDS CAN ENJOY DAIRY FREE DIET TOO 140

RECIPES: 141

DAIRY FREE BREAKFAST RECIPES 141

Applesauce.. 141
Buckwheat Walnut Muffins... 143
Pumpkin Spice Muffins 145
Milk Free Latte 147
Banana Nut Bread... 148
Basic Pancakes 149
Orange Banana Berry Pancakes.................................. 151
Breaded Pancakes 153
Crepes 155
Hot Cocoa.. 156
Granola Bars.. 157
Banbergo Smoothie 159
Banana Blueberry Smoothie 160
Breakfast Banana Smoothie.. 161

LUNCH AND SUPPER RECIPES 162

Pork (or Lamb) Barbecue Sandwiches 162
Chicken and Fruit Salad.. 163
Clam Chowder.. 165
Chicken Noodle Soup 167
Super Easy Vegetable Beef Soup 169
Cream of Chicken Soup 171
Potato Soup.. 172
Split Pea Soup.. 173
Grilled Garlic Shrimp 175
Beefy Cabbage Casserole 177
Rack of Lamb 179

Tuna Casserole 181
Mango and Tuna Steaks 183
Chicken Tortilla Soup 186
Salisbury Steak 188
Balsamic Vinegar Chicken 190
Honey Rolled Chicken Kabobs 192
Basic Fried Chicken 194
Coleslaw 196
Cream Corn 198
Mac and Cheese 200
Squash Soup 202
Chicken A La King 204
Lasagna 206
Cabbage Soup 208
"Cheesy" Vegetable Casserole 209
Sweet Potato Soup 212
Chicken and Dumplings 213
Turkey Burgers 215

SNACKS AND DESSERTS 217
Banana Coconut Honey Oat Bars................................217
Pumpkin Pie 219
Cheese Popcorn..221
Chocolate Pudding 222
Chocolate Rice Crispy Bars 223
Coconut Flavored Rice Pudding 225
Crunchy Oatmeal Cookies 226
Yellow Cake..228
Fudge..230
Apple Crumb Dessert..231

DAIRY FREE DIET CONCLUSION 233

Cholesterol Lowering Cookbooks Introduction

The lowering of cholesterol in your diet can achieve a number of different results. For one thing, you will find that employing a low cholesterol diet actually makes your body feel better, and even cures some of the most common ailments. It should be noted however that while it is said to reduce the symptoms of PMS, not everyone will experience the same results, and with that being the case, your mileage may vary. In spite of that, lowering your cholesterol is a must, but what happens if you need to cut the dairy out of your diet? Most will never consider doing this, but there is a good reason to, believe it or not. Lactose intolerance is a common ailment in people all over the world, and while it might not always cause the most severe problems, it can make someone rather uncomfortable. That being said, learning to cook with lactose intolerance in mind should be one of your primary concerns.

This condition is essentially the inability to digest lactose, which is a sugar found in milk. This also extends to milk based dairy products, though not so much. Rather than being a disorder, lactose intolerance is actually a genetic condition; you cannot control whether or not you suffer from it. With this condition, there is a severe lack of lactase, an enzyme in the body responsible for catalyzing hydrolysis. In most cases, consumption of lactose will cause anything from abdominal bloating, to flatulence and nausea. In addition to that, it has been concluded in scientific studies that significant milk consumption by those suffering from lactose intolerance can contribute to inflammatory bowel disease.

It should be noted that most mammals in the animal kingdom become lactose intolerant after being weaned from their mother's milk, but human beings have what is known as lactase persistence. 75% of adults have a decrease of lactase in their bodies during adulthood. The best way to cope with lactose intolerance of course is to try avoiding foods that contain dairy products. Many of the recipes contained within this book will help you to do just that, ensuring you have a great tasting diet while maintaining the maximum amount of comfort throughout your day. Remember, being lactose intolerant is nothing to be ashamed of! The majority of animals are lactose intolerant – as human beings, we are a bit of a natural phenomenon. That being said, using this cookbook will easily take you back to your natural roots whether you're lactose intolerant or not.

In addition to covering the concept of dairy free foods, this book will also take a close look at superfoods. What are superfoods exactly? You hear about them all the time, but you should note that it is not a term used by dieticians and food scientists. They, more often than not, tend to believe that the foods defined do not have the health benefits claimed by most individuals. The problem here is that there has been very little research, and as a result, there is a bit of a wide spectrum. One of the most common superfoods is blueberries, which have high levels of antioxidants.

Meal planning is yet another aspect of this book. How do you go about planning meals exactly? What is involved? If you happen to be new to the dieting, you might not know how to compose your own meals, or even how to judge the various calorie amounts. That being the case, it makes sense to have someone plan these meals for you. This book contains plans for every single time of day from the early morning to the late evening. Before you know it, you will be living the healthy life you have always dreamed of. It might sound like a dream, but let's be honest, when it comes to the state of your health, dreams can come true more often than not. You are in control of your body, and while it might be difficult to lose weight sometimes, you will not be stopped from making yourself feel healthier. More than a few people have embarked on a diet of this nature only to find that their energy increased and their quality of life improved astronomically. Yes, it will require some sacrifices on your part, but to be honest, it is quite worth it!

One of the final things this book covers is the concept of starting your children on this diet. Yes, this is an outstanding diet, but as you know, children are always growing, and their bodies might not be able to accept the change. Within this book you will find solutions for children, ensuring that they too can participate in this activity with you. Your entire family can participate of course, and you will find that it not only makes them feel healthier, but also improves their quality of life. The family that diets together, stays together, and they will have many extra years together that they might not have had otherwise. All diets are going to be work, of course, but soon enough, and with enough patience, you are going to find that all that work was well worth it.

While there are many fad diets out there that do not seem to pan out, or even cause harm to their users, these recipes are all natural and designed to give you the life you deserve. Start looking through this book today and create a new dietary routine for yourself. It might be difficult to stick with it at first, but as you progress, you will find it easier and easier to get where you want to be in life. That being said, it's time to embark on your journey, and if possible, take a few friends with you. There's nothing like having company, and it helps you stick with your chosen path. The ultimate diet and the ultimate lifestyle is finally within your grasp!

Section 1: Superfoods Introduction

Before we say anything else about superfoods and the recipes that you'll find in this book, it's important to mention that superfoods isn't a term which nutritionists or dieticians use. In fact, there isn't any single, universally accepted definition of the term, although it is used to market all manner of food products and nutritional supplements. That doesn't mean, however, that some foods aren't, for lack of a better term, super in terms of their nutritional value and health benefits.

Perhaps the most useful definition of superfoods is this: a food which is rich in essential nutrients, phytochemicals and other beneficial compounds, but that is also healthy in the broadest sense. These are fairly low calorie foods which contain no additives or artificial ingredients.

The best superfoods are also some of the easiest to find at your local market. Foods like pumpkin and other winter squashes, wild salmon, beans and lentils, spinach and other dark leafy greens, blueberries, kiwi fruit, oats, sweet potatoes and even chocolate (dark chocolate, not milk chocolate). Common though these foods may be, they all meet the superfoods criteria and are highly nutritious, healthy foods which deserve a prominent place in anyone's diet.

We'll go into the nutritional benefits of these superfoods in a little more detail in the individual chapters which follow. From vitamins and to phytonutrients which may play a role in preventing illness, to fiber and of course, flavor, these are foods which have a lot to offer your palate and your health.

Salmon

Salmon is the exception among superfoods in that it's an animal product rather than a fruit, vegetable or seed. Salmon is one of the richest sources of omega-3 fatty acids, a compound which can promote cognitive development, possibly improve mood and fight inflammation (and as such, is thought to help prevent certain forms of cancer as well as stroke and heart disease, among other illnesses). It's also an excellent source of lean protein and vitamin D, as well as carotenoid compounds (which are what give salmon its distinctive color).

One important thing to keep in mind when you're choosing salmon at your local market is to always opt for wild caught salmon. Farmed salmon will do in a pinch, but studies have shown that farmed salmon tends to contain lower levels of omega 3 fatty acids as well as having levels of PCB and dioxins which are as much as eight times higher than those found in their wild caught counterparts – as with any other food, it seems that the more natural your salmon is, the better it is for you.

Sweet Coconut Crusted Salmon

Number of servings: 4

Ingredients:

4 salmon filets, about 4 ounces each
1 cup butter
¾ cups coconut flakes
¾ cup honey

Preparation:

Place the butter in a small saucepan over medium heat. Melt the butter, then mix in the coconut flakes and honey once the butter has melted completely. Stir well to combine and bring to a boil, then remove from heat. Allow the mixture to cool slightly, then transfer to a large bowl. Add the salmon, turn to coat the fish with the butter, honey and coconut mixture, cover and refrigerate. Allow to marinate for at least 30 minutes while you preheat your oven to 375 F.

Pour a little of the marinade into a baking dish; just enough to coat the bottom. Place the salmon filets in the dish and pour marinade over the top, reserving a little for basting. Transfer the dish into the oven and bake for 25 minutes or until the salmon flakes easily with a fork, basting occasionally with the remaining marinade. Remove from the oven and serve hot.

Salmon Quiche

Number of servings: varies (recipe yields 1 9" quiche)

Ingredients:

1 lb wild salmon, cooked, deboned and flaked
1 9" pre-made pie crust
4 ounces sharp cheddar cheese, cubed
4 ounces sharp cheddar cheese, shredded
4 eggs
½ of a small red onion, diced
½ cup milk
½ tsp dried sage
½ tsp dried parsley
½ tsp garlic powder
salt and black pepper, to taste

Preparation:

Start by preheating your oven to 375 F. Add the eggs, onion, milk and cubed sharp cheddar cheese to a blender or food processor, along with the spices and a little salt and black pepper. Blend until smooth. Place the crust into a 9" pie tin and spread with flaked salmon. Top with half of the shredded cheddar cheese, then pour the egg mixture over the salmon and cheese, then top with the remaining shredded cheese. Transfer to the oven and bake for about 30 minutes, or until a toothpick inserted into the center of the quiche comes out clean. Remove from the oven and allow the quiche to cool for 5 minutes before slicing and serving.

Quick and Easy Pan Fried Salmon

Number of servings: 2

Ingredients:

2 salmon filets (with skin), about 4 ounces each
2 tbsp olive oil
salt and black pepper, to taste

Preparation:

Rinse the salmon filets well and pat dry with paper towels until excess moisture is removed. Season the filets with a little salt and black pepper. Set aside.

Heat the olive oil over medium high heat in a heavy skillet. Once the oil is hot, place it gently into the skillet, skin side up. Cook for 5 – 7 minutes or until the flesh side is golden brown. Turn the filets over and cook for another 5 minutes, or until the skin side is lightly browned. Remove the salmon from the skillet and transfer to a plate covered with paper towels to drain off any excess oil. Transfer to individual plates and serve hot.

Tunisian Style Baked Salmon

Number of servings: 4

Ingredients:

4 salmon filets, about 4 ounces each
2 thin slices of red onion, separated into rings
4 thin lemon slices (slices, not wedges)
¼ cup mayonnaise
1 tbsp dry white wine
1 tsp fresh lemon juice
2 tsp harissa, or more to taste*
1 tsp paprika (use smoked paprika if you can get it)
1 tsp canola oil
salt and black pepper, to taste

* Harissa is a North African hot sauce made from chili peppers, caraway and other spices. If you don't have a middle eastern market in your city, you can make a close approximation of harissa by adding a little bit of crushed garlic and ground caraway seed to Rooster or a similar Thai chili sauce. If you can find harissa in your city, however, the real thing is definitely preferable.

Preparation:

Start by preheating your oven to 425 F and lightly oil a large baking dish with canola oil. Season the salmon filets with a little salt and black pepper and transfer to the baking dish. Top the filets with onion and a lemon slice each. In a small bowl, mix together the mayonnaise, harissa, lemon juice and paprika, then mix until thoroughly combined. Spread the mixture over the fish, lemon and onion, then drizzle the wine over the top.

Transfer the salmon to the oven and bake until it begins to turn opaque (about 10 minutes), then turn on your broiler and broil for about 3 minutes or until the fish is nicely browned on top. Remove from the oven and serve hot.

Baked Salmon with Lemon and Dill

Number of servings: 4

Ingredients:

4 salmon filets, about 4 ounces each
¼ cup melted butter
juice of ½ lemon
1 tbsp dried dill
2 tsp crushed garlic (about 2 cloves)
salt and black pepper, to taste
cooking spray

Preparation:

Preheat your oven to 350 F and lightly coat a baking dish
with cooking spray. Place the salmon filets in the dish.
Whisk together the melted butter and lemon juice and
drizzle over the salmon, then top with the spices and a
little salt and pepper. Transfer the salmon to the oven
and bake for 25 minutes, or until the salmon easily
flakes with a fork. Remove from the oven and serve at
once.

Salmon Ceviche

Number of servings: 6

Ingredients:

1 lb high quality salmon filets, sliced thinly (use sushi-grade salmon if possible)
1 avocado, sliced thinly
1 tomato, diced small
2 cloves of garlic, minced
½ of a small red onion, minced
2 tbsp minced cilantro
¼ cup extra virgin olive oil
juice of 4 limes
2 tbsp salt
a pinch of cumin
a pinch of sugar
black pepper, to taste

Preparation:

Mix together the salt, sugar and lime juice in a large bowl, then stir in the cumin and black pepper. Add the remaining ingredients, gently mix to combine, cover and refrigerate for at least 4 hours or overnight to marinate.

Season to taste with black pepper before serving.

Salmon – Cream Cheese Dip

Number of servings: varies

Ingredients:

½ pound cooked salmon, skin and bones removed and flaked
8 ounces cream cheese, softened at room temperature
½ cup plain Greek yogurt
2 tbsp butter, softened at room temperature
2 tbsp diced pimentos
1 tbsp finely chopped Italian parsley
2 tsp minced red onion
1 tsp dill

Preparation:

Combine all of the ingredients in a bowl, except for the salmon. Blend until smooth with an electric mixer. Stir in the salmon, cover and refrigerate for a few hours or overnight.

Spinach

Spinach, like many other leafy greens, is one of those vegetables that many people hate as children and love as adults. Even if you don't think that you like spinach, the health benefits of this nutritional powerhouse alone merit another try – and when it's prepared as a part of delicious meals like these, you may well find that you like it after all!

Spinach is an excellent source of many vitamins, minerals and other nutrients, most notably vitamin C, vitamin K, foliate, zinc and selenium, as well as smaller amounts of protein, vitamin E, magnesium, niacin and omega-3 fatty acids, among others. Popeye was on to something, certainly and so were your parents; they weren't trying to be mean to you by making you eat your spinach as a child. If any food deserves the title of superfood, spinach certainly fits the bill.

Spinach is wonderful cooked in a variety of dishes, but like any other vegetable, you'll get the most benefit by eating it raw or very lightly cooked. The following recipes include a few such dishes, but either way, don't skip (or skimp on) this ultra nutritious leafy green!

Spinach, Lentil and Bean Curry

Number of servings: 4

Ingredients:

4 cups chopped fresh spinach, loosely packed
1 cup cooked kidney beans, drained and rinsed if using canned
1 cup dried red lentils
½ cup plain yogurt
2 medium sized tomatoes, diced
1 medium sized onion, diced
3 cloves of garlic, minced
1" piece of ginger, grated or crushed
¼ cup pureed tomatoes
2 tbsp chopped cilantro
2 tbsp canola oil
2 tsp garam masala
1 tsp turmeric
1 tsp cumin
1 tsp ancho chili powder
salt and black pepper, to taste

Preparation:

Rinse the lentils and place in a small saucepan with water to cover. Bring the lentils to a boil, then reduce heat to low, cover the saucepan and simmer for 20 minutes, or until the lentils are tender and have absorbed most of the water. Drain off any excess water and set aside.

Mix together the yogurt, tomato puree and spices in a bowl and combine well while heating the oil over medium heat in a large, heavy skillet. Add the garlic, ginger and onion and cook, stirring regularly until the onion starts to brown. Add the spinach and cook until just wilted, then stir in the yogurt mixture, cilantro and tomatoes. Add the cooked lentils and kidney beans, stir to combine and cook for 3 – 4 minutes or until the lentils and beans are heated through. Remove from heat and serve.

Beef Stew with Spinach

Number of servings: 6

Ingredients:

1 lb lean beef round, sliced thinly and cut into bite sized
pieces
2 bunches of fresh spinach, rinsed well, patted dry and
torn into 1" pieces
6 Roma tomatoes, diced
1 medium sized yellow onion, diced
4 small potatoes, quartered
4 cloves of garlic, minced
2 cups pureed tomato
1 ¾ cups beef broth
½ cup dry red wine
2 tbsp chopped fresh oregano
vegetable oil, for browning (about 1 tbsp)
salt and black pepper, to taste

Preparation:

Heat the vegetable oil in a skillet over medium high
heat. Add the beef and cook until well browned, then
transfer the beef to a stock pot. Add the onions and

garlic to the skillet and cook in the remaining oil and fat until tender and lightly browned, stirring occasionally. Add the tomatoes and cook until about half of the liquid has evaporated, then transfer the mixture to the stock pot along with the beef.

Add the potatoes to the skillet and brown over medium high heat, turning occasionally to brown all sides. Transfer the potatoes to the stock pot, along with the spinach, pureed tomato, red wine, garlic and oregano. Add the beef broth, bring to a boil, then reduce the heat to a simmer, cover and cook for about 1 hour. Season to taste with salt and black pepper and serve.

Curried Spinach and Chickpeas

Number of servings: 4

Ingredients:

1can (15 ounces) chickpeas, drained and rinsed (or 1 ½ cups homemade)
2 large bunches of fresh spinach, washed, stems removed
1 package (12 ounces) firm tofu, cubed
1 medium sized yellow onion, diced
2 cloves of garlic, minced or crushed
1 tbsp curry paste (your choice)
1 tbsp canola oil
salt and black pepper, to taste

Preparation:

Heat the oil in a large skillet or wok over medium heat; once the oil is hot, add the onions and sauté until translucent, stirring regularly. Add the curry paste and garlic and cook for 3 minutes, stirring occasionally. Add the chickpeas and tofu and stir gently. Reduce the heat slightly and cover. Cook, covered for 2 – 3 minutes or until the spinach is just wilted. Remove from heat, season to taste with salt and black pepper and serve.

Wilted Spinach Salad with Goat Cheese and Cherries

Number of servings: 4

Ingredients:

1 bag (10 ounces) baby spinach leaves
1 small red onion (or ½ of a medium sized onion), diced
2 cloves of garlic, minced
1 cup sliced crimini mushrooms
¼ cup dried tart cherries
2 tbsp crumbled goat cheese
1 tbsp olive oil
black pepper, to taste

Preparation:

Heat the olive oil over low heat in a large skillet. Add the onion, garlic, mushrooms and cherries and cook, stirring regularly, for about 5 minutes, or until the mushrooms and onions are tender but not browned. Add the spinach and cook until just wilted, about 3 minutes. Remove from heat, divide among individual plates and serve topped with a little goat cheese and black pepper.

Baked Spinach and Feta Pitas

Number of servings: 6

Ingredients:

6 whole wheat pitas (6" size)
2 Roma tomatoes, diced
1 bunch spinach, washed, patted dry and chopped
4 crimini mushrooms, sliced
6 ounces sun dried tomato pesto
½ cup crumbled feta cheese
3 tbsp olive oil
black pepper, to taste

Preparation:

Preheat your oven to 350 F while you prepare your pitas for baking. Spread each piece of pita with sun dried tomato pesto and place on a large baking sheet, pesto side up. Top the pitas with spinach, tomatoes, mushrooms and feta. Drizzle with a little olive oil and a sprinkling of black pepper.

Transfer the baking sheet to the oven and bake for 10 – 12 minutes, or until the pitas are crisp and the toppings are slightly browned. Slice each pita into quarters and serve immediately.

Chicken Florentine

Number of servings: 4

Ingredients:

4 chicken breast halves, skinless, boneless and sliced
into strips
8 ounces penne pasta, uncooked
2 cups loosely packed spinach leaves
2 cloves of garlic, minced
4 tbsp pesto
2 tbsp olive oil
1 tbsp grated Romano or Parmesan cheese

Preparation:

Heat the oil over medium high heat in a large skillet
while bringing water to a boil to cook the pasta. Once
the oil is hot, add the garlic and sauté for about 1 minute
or until it becomes fragrant. Add the chicken breasts and
cook for 7 – 8 minutes per side. When the chicken is
close to being cooked through, add the spinach and cook
for 3 – 4 minutes, or until just wilted. Reduce the heat to
low.

Once the pasta is finished, drain and rinse under cold water. Return to the pan. Add the chicken mixture, then the pesto. Stir well to combine, divide among individual plates and serve, topped with a little Romano or Parmesan cheese.

Fruit and Spinach Smoothie

Number of servings: 2

Ingredients:

1 banana, cut in half
1 cup of frozen grapes
½ apple, cored and diced
1 ½ cups baby spinach leaves
2/3 cup plain Greek yogurt

Preparation:

Place all of the ingredients in a blender and blend until smooth, stopping to push down anything which sticks to the side of the blender. Transfer into glasses and serve.

Quinoa

Quinoa may be a relative newcomer to the North American diet, but it's been a staple in the cuisine of the Andes for millennia now. This plant, a relative of beets rather than an actual grain, is grown for its seeds, which closely resemble grains in taste and more or less play the same role as rice in many other cuisines. Quinoa provides a complete protein as well as being rich in magnesium, phosphorus, potassium and B vitamins.

Try quinoa in the place of rice or other grains, as a breakfast porridge, as a base for salads and anywhere else that your culinary creativity takes you – these recipes don't cover all the bases, but they make a great introduction to this versatile and highly nutritious seed.

Baked Quinoa Breakfast Cereal

Number of servings: 2 – 3

Ingredients:

1 cup quinoa
¼ cup flax seed
1 tbsp canola oil
2 tbsp maple syrup
1 tsp cinnamon
cooking spray

Preparation:

Preheat your oven to 350 F and lightly coat a baking sheet with cooking spray. Rinse the quinoa well and drain thoroughly (unless you're using quinoa which has been pre-rinsed), then add to a large bowl with the rest of the ingredients. Stir until well combined and spread out the mixture on the baking sheet, forming as thin of a layer as possible. Bake until golden brown, about 15 – 17 minutes, stirring every 5 minutes. Remove from the oven and allow it to cool completely before serving. This can be stored in a covered airtight container once it has cooled to room temperature.

Five Spice Quinoa

Number of servings: 4

Ingredients:

2 cups water
1 cup quinoa, rinsed and drained
1 beef bouillon cube
1 ½ tbsp butter
1 tbsp five spice powder
½ tsp powdered ginger
black pepper, to taste

Preparation:

Place all of the ingredients except for the quinoa in a saucepan and bring to a boil, stirring until the bouillon cube is dissolved. Add the quinoa, reduce the heat to a simmer, cover and cook for about 20 minutes or until the quinoa has absorbed all of the liquid and is tender.

Quinoa Pilaf

Number of servings: 4

Ingredients:

1 cup quinoa, rinsed and drained
1 small yellow onion, diced
2 medium sized carrots, diced
2 cups vegetable stock
¾ cup chopped walnuts
¼ cup chopped Italian parsley
1 tbsp olive oil
salt and black pepper, to taste

Preparation:

Heat the olive oil in a saucepan over medium high heat. Once the oil is hot, add the onion and cook until translucent, stirring occasionally. Add the carrots and cook for another 3 minutes. Add the vegetable stock and quinoa and bring the mixture to a boil. Reduce the heat to a simmer, cover and cook for 15 – 20 minutes, or until the quinoa has absorbed all of the liquid and is tender. Transfer the cooked quinoa mixture to a bowl and toss with the parsley and walnuts. Season to taste with salt

and black pepper; serve at once or allow to cool and
serve at room temperature.

Quinoa and Mushrooms

Number of servings: 6

Ingredients:

1 ½ cups quinoa, rinsed
3 cups chicken broth
1 cup sliced crimini or button mushrooms
1 small yellow onion, diced
3 cloves of garlic, minced
1/3 cup grated Parmesan or Romano cheese
1 tbsp butter
1 tbsp olive oil
salt and black pepper, to taste

Preparation:

Heat the olive oil over medium heat in a large skillet. Add the mushrooms, garlic and onion to the hot oil and cook for about 5 minutes or until browned, stirring occasionally. Set aside.

Melt the butter in a saucepan over medium heat. Add the quinoa and brown, stirring regularly (this will take about 3 minutes). Add the chicken broth and bring the quinoa to a boil. Reduce the heat to low, cover and cook for about 15 minutes, or until the broth is almost absorbed. Add the mushroom mixture and cook for another 2 minutes, or until all of the broth is absorbed and the mushrooms are heated through. Season to taste with salt and black pepper, divide among individual plates and serve hot, topped with Parmesan or Romano cheese.

Broccoli and Quinoa Soup

Number of servings: 6

Ingredients:

2 cups of broccoli florets
2 cups chicken or vegetable broth
1 cup quinoa, rinsed
1 cup evaporated (not condensed) milk
½ of a medium sized yellow or white onion, diced
4 cloves of garlic, minced
1 tbsp flour
1 tbsp olive oil
salt and black pepper, to taste

Preparation:

Heat the olive oil over medium heat in a large skillet. Add the garlic and onion and cook until translucent, about 5 minutes, stirring regularly. Add the quinoa, broccoli and chicken or vegetable broth and bring to a boil. Cover, reduce the heat to low and simmer for 10 – 15 minutes, or until the quinoa is tender and fluffy and most of the liquid has been absorbed.

Add the flour and evaporated milk and bring the mixture back to a boil. Cook until the soup thickens, stirring constantly. Season to taste with salt and black pepper, divide among individual bowls and serve hot.

Quinoa Salad with Cranberries and Cilantro

Number of servings: 6

Ingredients:

1 cup quinoa, rinsed
1 ½ cups water
1 small red onion, diced small
¼ cup each diced red and yellow bell pepper
½ cup carrots, diced small
½ cup dried cranberries
¼ cup chopped cilantro
¼ cup toasted slivered almonds
1 ½ tsp curry powder (or more to taste)
juice of 1 lime
salt and black pepper, to taste

Preparation:

Bring the water to a boil in a covered saucepan. Add the quinoa, cover and reduce the heat to a summer. Cook for 15 – 20 minutes, or until the water has been absorbed and the quinoa is tender and fluffy. Transfer the cooked quinoa to a large mixing bowl and place in the refrigerator to chill. Once the quinoa is cold, stir in the remaining ingredients, season to taste with salt and black pepper and refrigerate before serving cold.

Beans and Lentils

Beans have something of a bad reputation due to their propensity to cause gas in many people, especially those who are unaccustomed to including them in their diet regularly. While there is no getting around this effect to some degree, beans are so nutritious that even this is no reason to avoid them entirely. When prepared properly and incorporated as a regular part of your diet, you'll find their less desirable effects greatly reduced and you'll enjoy their nutritional and health benefits in the bargain.

Beans and lentils are rich in protein, being perhaps the single best vegetarian source of this essential nutrient. They're also a natural choice for anyone trying to lose excess weight or maintain their weight, since they're a naturally high fiber food. As we all know, fiber plays an essential role in regulating digestion and appetite, since fiber helps you stay feeling full for longer, which curbs the urge to snack or to overeat at meals. They're also one of the best kinds of carbohydrates to include in your diet. Refined carbs may have earned their bad reputation, but natural carbohydrates like those found in beans, vegetables and fruit are the kind that you want to include in your diet.

Vegetarian Chili

Number of servings: 8

Ingredients:

1 can (15 ounces) each of black beans, chickpeas and kidney beans, drained and rinsed – or 1 ½ cups each of homemade cooked beans
1 ½ cups corn kernels (frozen and thawed or fresh cut from the cob)
1 medium sized yellow or white onion, diced
2 green bell peppers, diced
2 stalks of celery, diced
6 cloves of garlic, minced
2 – 3 jalapeno peppers, diced
3 large cans (10 ½ cups total) of crushed tomatoes
2 (4 ounce) cans of green chilies
1 tbsp olive oil
2 tbsp oregano
2 tbsp chili powder (your choice)
1 tbsp cumin
1 tbsp salt, or to taste
1 tbsp black pepper, or to taste
2 bay leaves

Preparation:

Heat the olive oil over medium heat in a stock pot. Once the oil is hot, add the onion, oregano, cumin, bay leaves and salt. Cook until the onion turns translucent, stirring regularly. Add the peppers, garlic, celery and green chilies and cook for 3 -4 minutes, stirring occasionally. Reduce the heat to low, cover and simmer the vegetables and spices for 5 minutes.

Add the tomatoes, chili powder, black pepper and beans. Bring the chili to a boil, then reduce the heat to low, cover and simmer for 45 minutes. Add the corn, stir and cook for another 5 minutes to heat through before serving.

Pasta Fagioli

Number of servings: 8

Ingredients:

1 (15 ounce) can cannellini beans or 1 ½ cups
homemade cannellini beans
1 (15 ounce) can navy beans or 1 ½ cups homemade
navy beans
1 lb ditalini
1 large yellow or white onion, diced
4 cloves of garlic, minced
1 large (28 ounce) can pureed tomato
5 ½ cups water
3 tbsp olive oil
1 tbsp dried parsley
2 tsp each dried oregano and basil
1/3 cup grated Romano or Parmesan cheese
salt and black pepper, to taste

Preparation:

Heat the olive oil in a large saucepan or stock pot over
medium heat and cook the onion until translucent,
stirring occasionally. Add the garlic and cook until

fragrant, about 2 minutes. Reduce the heat to medium low and add the remaining ingredients except for the ditalini and cheese. Simmer for 1 hour.

Bring lightly salted water to a boil in another large pot and cook the ditalini until al dente. Drain the pasta and stir it into the soup. Season to taste with salt and black pepper and serve hot.

Cuban Style Black Beans

Number of servings: 12

Ingredients:

2 cups dry black beans, soaked overnight
1 medium to large yellow onion, diced
1 green bell pepper, diced
6 cloves of garlic, chopped
½ cup dry white wine
¼ cup olive oil
2 tbsp white or apple cider vinegar
1 tbsp salt, or to taste
1 tbsp black pepper, or to taste
1 tbsp cumin
1 tbsp oregano
2 bay leaves

Preparation:

Add the black beans to a stock pot with enough water to cover plus 2". Add the onion, green pepper, garlic, salt, cumin, oregano and bay leaves. Bring to a boil, then reduce the heat to a simmer and cook, covered for 1 -2 hours, adding water as necessary to prevent the beans from drying out or burning. When the beans are nearly done, add the wine, oil and vinegar and stir well. Continue cooking uncovered until the alcohol cooks off, remove from heat and serve.

Black Bean Hummus

Number of servings: 8

Ingredients:

1 (15 ounce) can of black beans, drained and rinsed (or 1 ½ cups homemade)
2 cloves of garlic, minced
2 tbsp water
2 tbsp tahini
juice of 1 lemon
1 tsp cumin
½ tsp salt
¼ tsp cayenne pepper, or more to taste
¼ tsp paprika

Preparation:

Add the black beans, garlic, water, lemon juice, tahini, cumin, salt and cayenne pepper to a food processor. Blend until smooth, adding additional water as needed. Transfer to a bowl, sprinkle with paprika and serve at once or chill until ready to serve.

Southwestern Breakfast Platter

Number of servings: 2

Ingredients:

1 (15 ounce) can of black beans, drained and rinsed (or 1 ½ cup homemade)
4 eggs, beaten
1 avocado, peeled, seeded and sliced
¼ cup salsa (your choice), or more to taste
2 tbsp olive oil
salt and black pepper, to taste

Preparation:

Heat the olive oil in a small skillet over medium heat. Add the eggs and cook until set, about 3 minutes. While the eggs are cooking, microwave the beans for about minute or until hot. Divide the beans between two bowls and top each with eggs, avocado slices and salsa. Season to taste with salt and black pepper and serve immediately.

Lentil Soup

Number of servings: 8

Ingredients:

1 ½ cups lentils, soaked, rinsed and drained
3 ½ cups crushed tomatoes
2 celery stalks, diced
2 cloves garlic, minced
1 large onion, diced
2 medium sized carrots, diced
1 sprig of Italian parsley, chopped
7 cups chicken or vegetable stock
¾ cup dry white wine
½ cup grated Romano or Parmesan cheese
2 tbsp olive oil
1 tsp paprika
2 bay leaves
salt and black pepper, to taste

Preparation:

Heat the oil in a stockpot and sauté the onions until they turn translucent. Add the garlic, carrots, celery and paprika and cook for 10 minutes, stirring occasionally.

Add the tomatoes, chicken or vegetable stock and bay leaves. Stir and add the wine, then bring to a boil. Reduce the heat to a simmer and cook, covered for 1 hour or until the lentils are tender. Season to taste with salt and black pepper and serve, topped with chopped parsley and Romano or Parmesan cheese.

Baked Chicken and Lentils

Number of servings: 6

Ingredients:

2 lbs chicken, bone-in
1 ¾ cups chicken or vegetable broth
1 ¼ cups tomato sauce or pureed tomato
¾ cup dried lentils
1 large onion, diced
1 small carrot, diced
4 cloves of garlic, minced
juice of ½ lemon
1 tbsp olive oil
1 tsp rosemary
1 tsp basil
salt and black pepper, to taste

Preparation:

Heat the olive oil over medium heat in a large, heavy skillet. Once the oil is hot, cook the chicken pieces for 5 minutes per side or until the juices run clear and the chicken is lightly browned on both sides. Remove from the skillet and set aside. Add the onion to the skillet and cook until tender, stirring occasionally, then add the garlic, carrots and sauté for another 5 minutes, stirring occasionally.

Add the lentils and broth and bring to a boil, then reduce to a simmer, cover and cook for about 20 minutes. Return the chicken to the skillet and cook for another 20 minutes, adding a little water if necessary. Add the tomato sauce, rosemary and basil and stir. Once the lentils are tender, add the lemon juice, stir well and serve hot.

Apples

Apples may not contain the nutritional cornucopia that some other fruits and vegetables have to offer, but there's a lot to recommend these sweet, crisp and almost universally loved fruits. Their high fiber content and antioxidant content make them a natural health food – and studies suggest that an apple a day really may keep the doctor away. The regular consumption of apples has been linked to a lower risk of colon, lung and prostate cancers, as well as helping to control cholesterol levels and assisting in weight loss.

While apples are usually thought of as an ingredient in desserts and indeed, there are some dessert recipes for apples in this book, they're also a good fit for savory dishes where their sweetness plays off of the flavors of other ingredients and as a component of salads. Apples are great eaten out of hand, but it's well worth experimenting with using them in your cooking.

Apple Soup

Number of servings: 4

Ingredients:

2 Granny Smith apples, peeled, cored and cubed
1 small russet potato, cubed (peeling optional)
2 shallots, minced
2 tsp grated or crushed ginger
3 ¾ cups chicken or vegetable stock
½ cup heavy cream
2 tbsp curry powder
1 tbsp butter
salt and black pepper, to taste
plain Greek yogurt, for garnish

Preparation:

Melt the butter in a large saucepan over medium heat. Add the shallots and sauté until translucent. Add the curry powder and ginger and cook for 1 minute, stirring regularly. Add the apples, potato and chicken or vegetable stock. Bring the soup to a simmer and cook until the potato is tender. Remove from heat and allow the soup to cool slightly before transferring to a blender.

Blend until smooth and return to the pan. Add the cream and season to taste with salt and black pepper. Cook for a few minutes to heat through. Divide among individual bowls and serve hot, garnished with a dollop of plain yogurt.

Brown Rice Salad with Fruit and Nuts

Number of servings: 6 - 8

2 cups cooked brown rice, cooled to room temperature
3/4 cup fresh or frozen peas (thaw first if using frozen)
1 apple, diced
1/4 cup dried cherries, chopped
1/3 cup walnuts, chopped
1 bunch of chives, chopped
The dressing:
2 cloves of garlic, minced
2 tbsp miso paste
2 tbsp toasted sesame seeds
2 tbsp canola oil
2 tbsp balsamic vinegar or red wine vinegar
1 tbsp honey

Preparation:

Combine all of the ingredients for the salad in a large
bowl. Whisk together the ingredients for the dressing.
Stir the dressing into the salad, mixing well to coat.
Garnish with chives and sesame seeds and refrigerate,
covered, overnight to allow the flavors to blend.

Braised Escarole

Number of servings: 4

Ingredients:

10 cups roughly chopped escarole
1 large apple (your choice), cored and cut into wedges
(peeling optional)
2 strips of bacon
salt and black pepper, to taste

Preparation:

Cook the bacon over medium heat in a large skillet until crisp. Remove and place on paper towels to drain. Add the apples and escarole to the skillet and toss to coat with the bacon grease. Season with a little salt and black pepper, reduce the heat to a simmer and cook, covered for 8 – 10 minutes or until the escarole is dark green and wilted. Serve hot topped with crumbled bacon and salt and black pepper to taste.

Apple Coleslaw

Number of servings: 6

Ingredients:

4 cups shredded cabbage
1 cup shredded carrot
1 Granny Smith apple, cored and shredded
2 tbsp honey
2 tbsp mayonnaise
2 tsp white vinegar or apple cider vinegar
salt and black pepper, to taste

Preparation:

Mix the cabbage, carrot and apple in a bowl and toss to combine. In a separate small bowl, whisk together the mayonnaise, honey and vinegar. Pour over the salad, toss to coat, season to taste with salt and black pepper, toss again, cover and chill until you're ready to serve the coleslaw.

Apple Chutney

Number of servings: varies (recipe yields about 5 cups)

Ingredients:

15 tart apples - peeled, cored, and diced small
1 yellow onion, diced
3 small (1") pieces of fresh ginger, peeled
1 cup white wine or apple cider vinegar
½ cup brown sugar
1 tsp white pepper
1 tsp cinnamon
1 tsp cardamom
½ tsp nutmeg

Preparation:

Mix together all of the ingredients in a saucepan and bring to a boil. Reduce heat and simmer, covered for 30 minutes, uncovering and stirring occasionally, or until the apples are very tender, adding a little extra water as needed. Remove from heat, remove the ginger and transfer to a bowl. Cover and refrigerate until you're ready to serve your chutney.

Apple Turnovers

Number of servings: 8

Ingredients:

4 Granny Smith apples, cored and sliced (peeling optional)
4 cups water
1 cup brown sugar
2 tbsp lemon juice
2 tbsp butter
1 tbsp water
1 tsp corn starch
1 tsp cinnamon
1 package (17.25 ounces) frozen puff pastry sheets, thawed
The icing:
1 cup powdered sugar
1 tbsp milk
1 tsp vanilla extract

Preparation:

Add the lemon juice, water and sliced apples to a large bowl (the lemon juice will prevent the apples from browning). Melt the butter over medium heat in a large skillet. Once the butter is melted, drain the apples and transfer to the skillet. Cook for about 2 minutes, stirring regularly. Add the sugar and cinnamon and continue cooking for another 2 minutes, stirring occasionally. Mix the water and corn starch and add to the skillet. Mix well and cook until the sauce thickens, about 1 minute. Remove from heat and allow it to cool slightly.

While the filling cools, preheat your oven to 400 F. Unfold the pastry sheets and trim each into a square, then divide into 4 roughly equal squares. Spoon filling onto the center of each square, then fold over into a triangle shape, pressing the edges to seal. Place the turnovers on a baking sheet, leaving a little space in between. Bake for 25 minutes or until they're lightly browned and puffed up. Remove the turnovers from the oven and allow them to cool to room temperature. Make the glaze by mixing together the sugar, milk and vanilla extract, then drizzle over the turnovers before serving.

Apple Crisp

Number of servings: 12

Ingredients:

10 cups sliced apples
2 cups brown sugar
1 cup oats
½ cup water
½ cup melted butter
1 cup plus 1 tbsp all purpose flour
1 tsp cinnamon
¼ tsp baking soda
¼ tsp baking powder

Preparation:

Start by preheating your oven to 350 F. Arrange the sliced apples in a large (9" x 13") baking pan. Mix together 1 cup of the brown sugar, 1 tbsp flour and 1 tsp cinnamon, then sprinkle over the apples, then pour water evenly over the ingredients in the baking pan.

In a bowl, mix together the oats, the melted butter, baking soda, baking powder and the remaining flour and brown sugar. Layer the mixture evenly over the apples. Transfer the baking pan to the oven and bake for about 45 minutes or until the top is golden brown. Remove from the oven and allow the apple crisp to cool slightly before serving.

Yogurt

In ancient India, yogurt was referred to as the food of the gods; and medieval Persian tradition held that the longevity ascribed to the prophet Abraham by the Bible and the Qur'an was due to his regular consumption of yogurt. While yogurt may not be divine as such, it certainly is healthy, delicious and deserves a place in your diet.

Yogurt contains lactobacilli and/or acidophilus, helpful bacteria which can improve digestion; in fact, even people who are otherwise lactose intolerant can often eat yogurt and enjoy its nutritional benefits. Additionally, plain yogurt, especially Greek style yogurt, is a good source of protein and calcium. It has been suggested by some studies that eating low fat yogurt regularly can also help to promote weight loss. Just remember to steer clear of fruit flavored, sweetened yogurt – if you want fruit in your yogurt, add fresh fruit to some plain yogurt. It's even more delicious and you won't miss the added sugar at all!

Yogurt Pound Cake

Number of servings: varies (recipe yields 1 10" bundt pan)

Ingredients:

2 ¼ cups all purpose flour
1 cup plain Greek yogurt
1 cup margarine, softened at room temperature (butter may be substituted)
1 ½ cups white or turbinado sugar
3 eggs
½ tsp salt
½ tsp baking soda
juice of 1 lemon
cooking spray

Preparation:

Preheat your oven to 325 F. Lightly coat the inside of a 10" bundt pan with cooking spray, then flour. Sift the flour, salt and baking soda and set aside. Cream the margarine (or butter) and sugar in a bowl, then beat in the eggs, one at a time. Add the lemon juice, then add the wet ingredient mixture and yogurt to the flour mixture, stirring just until incorporated.

Pour the batter into your prepared bundt pan and bake for 1 hour, or until a toothpick inserted into the center comes out clean. Remove from the oven and allow the cake to cool in the pan for about 10 minutes, then turn the cake out onto a wire rack and cool to room temperature before serving.

Yogurt Rice

Number of servings: 8 (about 4 cups)

Ingredients:

1 cup jasmine rice
2 cups water
1 cup plain yogurt
¼ cup milk
1 dried red chili pepper or more to taste, broken into a
few pieces
1 tbsp ghee (clarified butter)
1 tsp mustard seeds (preferably black mustard seeds)
1 tsp turmeric
½ tsp asafoetida
4 curry leaves (may be omitted if you can't find these)
salt, to taste

Preparation:

Cook the rice in 2 cups water until tender. Keep covered
and set aside. In a small skillet, heat the ghee over
medium heat and add the chili pepper. Cook for about
30 seconds, or until fragrant, then add the mustard
seeds and cook for another 30 seconds or until they

begin to pop. Remove from heat and add the curry leaves, asafetida and turmeric. Transfer the spices and ghee to a large bowl and whisk together with the yogurt and milk. Fold in the cooked rice and stir well to mix. Allow the rice to cool to room temperature, season to taste with salt and serve.

Beet and Yogurt Salad

Number of servings: 2

Ingredients:

2 cups plain yogurt
1 ½ cups cooked beets, peeled, sliced and cooled to
room temperature
2 tbsp chopped cilantro
1 tbsp canola oil
½ tsp black mustard seeds
½ tsp cumin seeds
salt and black pepper, to taste

Preparation:

Heat the oil over medium heat in a skillet; once the oil is
hot, add the mustard seeds and cook until they begin to
pop, about 30 seconds. Add the cumin seeds, cook for
another 30 seconds, then remove from heat.

Mix the yogurt and beets in a large bowl, then add the
mustard and cumin seeds. Season to taste with salt and
black pepper, stir, sprinkle with the chopped cilantro
and serve.

Yogurt Chicken

Number of servings: 4 – 6

Ingredients:

4 skinless, boneless chicken breasts
1 cup plain yogurt
1 cup seasoned bread crumbs
¼ cup butter
juice of 1 lemon
1 tbsp chopped Italian parsley
1 tsp garlic powder
salt and black pepper, to taste

Preparation:

Preheat your oven to 350 F. Add the yogurt to a small bowl and stir well until smooth, then add the lemon juice and stir again. Mix together the bread crumbs, garlic powder and a little salt and pepper in a shallow dish.

Place 1 pat of butter for each chicken breast in a 9" x 13" baking dish. Rinse the chicken and pat dry with paper towels. Dip each chicken breast in the yogurt mixture, then roll in the bread crumb mixture to coat lightly. Place the coated chicken breasts in the dish and top each with another pat of butter. Sprinkle with parsley and bake for 1 hour. Remove from the oven and allow the chicken to cool for at least 5 minutes before serving.

Yogurt Parfait with Blueberries

Number of servings: 2

Ingredients:

2 cups plain yogurt
4 graham crackers, crushed
1 cup fresh blueberries

Preparation:

Spoon half of the yogurt into the bottom of 2 parfait glasses. Layer half of the graham crackers on top of the yogurt, followed by half of the blueberries. Repeat the layering process and transfer the parfaits to the refrigerator to chill before serving.

Haydari

Number of servings: 8

Ingredients:

2 cups plain yogurt
5 cloves of garlic, crushed
a pinch of salt
4 tbsp fresh dill, chopped
1 bunch of Italian parsley, stems removed and chopped
mint leaves, for garnish (optional)

Preparation:

Place two layers of cheesecloth in a colander placed over a medium sized bowl. Place the yogurt in the colander and cover the colander with plastic wrap. Allow the yogurt to drain for 8 hours. Transfer the drained yogurt to a large bowl, then mix in the crushed garlic, salt, dill and parsley. Stir well to combine, then transfer into a serving dish. Chill briefly and serve cool, garnished with mint leaves if desired.

Eggplant and Yogurt Salad

Number of servings: 4

Ingredients:

1 medium sized eggplant, cubed
1 bunch of scallions, trimmed and sliced
½ of a small bunch of cilantro, stems removed and
chopped finely
1 ½ cups plain yogurt
½ cup water
1 tsp smoked paprika
salt and black pepper, to taste

Preparation:

Add the eggplant and water to a saucepan over medium
heat. Cook until the water is evaporated and the
eggplant is very tender. Mash with a fork to eliminate
any large pieces and allow the eggplant to cool to room
temperature. When the eggplant is cool, transfer to a
large bowl with the scallions, cilantro, smoked paprika
and yogurt and mix well to combine. Season to taste
with salt and black pepper, stir again, sprinkle with the
chopped cilantro, cover and refrigerate to chill before

serving – this salad can also be served at room temperature, if desired.

Yogurt Salad Dressing

Number of servings: varies (recipe yields about 1 cup)

Ingredients:

1 cup plain yogurt
2 tsp fresh lemon juice
1 tsp Dijon mustard
1 tsp chopped Italian parsley
1 teaspoon chopped fresh chives

Preparation:

Beat the lemon juice and yogurt together until smooth. Add the mustard, chives and parsley, stir to mix well, then cover and refrigerate until you're ready to use the dressing.

Spinach Dip with Yogurt

Number of servings: varies (recipe yields about 3 cups)

Ingredients:

1 cup plain yogurt
1 cup fresh spinach, chopped
½ cup mayonnaise
2 tsp salt
1 tsp dried parsley
¼ tsp basil
¼ tsp oregano
¼ tsp dry mustard
¼ tsp garlic powder, or more to taste
black pepper, to taste

Preparation:

Mix together all of the ingredients in a medium sized bowl, stirring well to combine. Cover and chill until ready to serve.

Turkish-Style Zucchini Salad

Number of servings: 4

Ingredients:

2 zucchini, grated
2 cups plain yogurt
2 tablespoons chopped walnuts
2 tbsp olive oil
salt and black pepper, to taste

Preparation:

Heat the olive oil over high heat in a skillet. Add the zucchini and cook for about 3 minutes, stirring constantly. Remove from heat and allow the zucchini to cool to room temperature. Mix the cooled zucchini with the yogurt and walnuts and season to taste with salt and black pepper. Cover and refrigerate until ready to serve.

Sweet Potatoes

There is an interesting and little known fact about this ultra-nutritious member of the morning glory family (despite the name, they're not related to potatoes, nor are they the same as yams, which are an unrelated root vegetable commonly eaten in Africa and the Caribbean): they're the only food which provides all of the essential nutrients the human body needs. You literally could eat nothing but sweet potatoes and still meet all of your nutritional requirements – although you'd probably get sick of sweet potatoes pretty fast!

While it's not necessary to go on an all sweet potato diet, these starchy tubers are delicious and nutritious enough that they should show up at your dinner table regularly. They're an especially good source of vitamin A and beta carotene, but this is a vegetable which truly has a little bit of everything and is adaptable enough to be perfect in both savory and sweet dishes.

Sweet and Spicy Sweet Potatoes

Number of servings: 4

Ingredients:

2 large sweet potatoes, cubed (peeling optional)
3 tbsp olive oil
1 tbsp paprika
2 tsp brown sugar
1 tsp garlic powder
1 tsp onion powder
1 tsp poultry seasoning
½ tsp chili powder
½ tsp cayenne pepper, or more to taste
salt and black pepper, to taste

Preparation:

Start by preheating your oven to 425 F. In a large mixing bowl, mix together all of the ingredients and toss to coat. Spread the sweet potatoes in a single layer on a baking sheet. Bake for 15 minutes, then turn and bake for another 15 minutes or until tender and golden brown.

Sweet Potato Soup

Number of servings: 8

Ingredients:

2 large sweet potatoes, peeled and cubed
1 medium sized yellow onion, sliced
2 cloves of garlic, sliced thin
1 Roma tomato, diced
4 cups chicken or vegetable stock
½ cup plain yogurt
¼ cup peanut butter
2 tbsp chopped cilantro
2 tbsp grated ginger
1 tbsp butter
1 tsp cumin
1 tsp crushed red pepper flakes
juice of 1 lime
zest of ½ lime
salt and black pepper, to taste

Preparation:

Mix the yogurt and lime zest in a bowl, then refrigerate.
Melt the butter in a large saucepan over medium heat.

Add the garlic and onion and cook until softened, stirring occasionally. Add the sweet potatoes and the chicken or vegetable stock, the cumin, ginger and crushed red pepper. Bring the mixture to a boil, then reduce to a simmer and cook, covered, for about 15 minutes or until the sweet potatoes are tender.

Transfer the soup to a blender and blend until smooth – you'll probably need to do this in batches. Return the pureed soup to the saucepan and whisk in the peanut butter and lime juice. Heat through, season to taste with salt and black pepper and serve hot garnished with diced tomato, chopped cilantro and a dollop of the yogurt and lime zest mixture.

Sweet Potato Rolls

Number of servings: 18 rolls

Ingredients:

3 ½ cups all purpose flour
½ cup pureed sweet potato
½ cup warm water
3 tbsp butter, softened at room temperature
2 tbsp sugar
2 eggs, lightly beaten
1 tsp salt
1 package active dry yeast

Preparation:

Dissolve the yeast and half of the sugar in warm water in a large mixing bowl; allow to stand for 5 minutes. Add the sweet potato, the rest of the sugar, the butter, salt and eggs and mix well. Add 3 cups of the flour, stir and turn out the dough onto a lightly floured work surface. Knead for a few minutes, adding a little extra flour as needed to prevent the dough from getting too sticky. Shape the dough into a ball and place in a lightly oiled bowl. Cover with a clean kitchen towel and set in a warm place to rise for at least 1 hour or until doubled in bulk.

Punch down the dough and allow it to rest for 2 -3 minutes before dividing into 18 roughly equally sized balls. Place on a lightly greased baking sheet, cover and allow the rolls to rise until they double in size; this is a good time to preheat your oven. Bake for 15 – 20 minutes, remove from the oven and serve warm.

Oven Roasted Sweet Potatoes

Number of servings: 6

Ingredients:

2 large sweet potatoes, cubed
2 medium sized sweet onions, diced into 1" pieces
¼ cup toasted sliced or slivered almonds
3 tbsp olive oil
2 tbsp amaretto (optional)
1 tsp thyme
salt and black pepper, to taste

Preparation:

Heat your oven to 425 F. Toss all of the ingredients except for the almonds in a baking dish to combine. Cover with foil and bake for 30 minutes. Uncover and bake for 10 minutes, then sprinkle with the almonds and bake for another 10 minutes. Remove from heat, season to taste with salt and black pepper and serve hot.

Sweet Potato Chili

Number of servings: 8

Ingredients:

½ lb lean ground beef
½ lb lean ground turkey
2 sweet potatoes, diced
1 small sweet onion, diced (about 2/3 – ¾ cup)
2 small celery stalks, diced
1 large can (28 ounces) diced tomatoes
1 ½ cups cooked or canned black beans, drained and
rinsed if using canned
1 cup tomato sauce or pureed tomato
1 cup fresh or frozen corn kernels (thaw first if using
frozen)
½ cup water
1 tsbp hot chili powder
1 tsp cumin
1 tsp each garlic powder and onion powder
½ tsp cinnamon
salt, black pepper and cayenne pepper, to taste

Preparation:

Place the tomatoes, tomato sauce, sweet potatoes, onion, celery, water and spices in a slow cooker set on high. Cook for 5 hours, stirring occasionally. Brown the ground beef and ground turkey in a skillet over medium high heat; drain off any excess fat. Add the cooked meat, beans and corn to the ingredients in the slow cooker and continue cooking for another 1 -2 hours to allow the flavors to combine. Season to taste with salt, black pepper and cayenne pepper and serve hot.

Sweet Potato Pie

Number of servings: varies (1 9" pie)

Ingredients:

1 9" unbaked pie crust, your choice
2 cups mashed sweet potatoes
¾ cup brown sugar
¾ cup milk
½ cup whipping cream
2 eggs, beaten
2 tbsp melted butter
1 tsp vanilla extract
1 tsp nutmeg
juice of 1 lemon

Preparation:

Start by preheating your oven to 375 F. Mix together the mashed sweet potatoes and melted butter in a large mixing bowl, then add the beaten eggs, brown sugar, milk, lemon juice, vanilla extract, whipping cream and nutmeg. Beat well until the mixture is smooth and then pour into the pie shell. Bake the pie for 50 – 60 minutes, or until a toothpick inserted into the center of the pie comes out clean. Serve warm or refrigerate and serve chilled.

Spicy Roasted Sweet Potatoes

Number of servings: 4

Ingredients:

4 sweet potatoes, cubed
6 tbsp olive oil
2 tsp cayenne pepper or more to taste
salt and black pepper, to taste

Preparation:

Preheat your oven to 375 F. Place all of the ingredients in a large re-sealable freezer bag and shake to coat. Transfer the coated sweet potatoes to a large baking dish and arrange in a single layer. Bake for about 1 hour or until the sweet potatoes are tender, stirring a few times during baking.

Sweet Potato Fries

Number of servings: 4

Ingredients:

2 large sweet potatoes, cut into French fry-size pieces
1 tbsp olive oil or more, if needed
2 tbsp fresh rosemary, minced
salt and black pepper, to taste

Preparation:

Preheat your oven to 425 F while you prepare the sweet potatoes. Toss all of the ingredients together in a large bowl to coat and arrange the fries in a single layer on a baking sheet. Bake until tender and slightly crisp on the outside, 25 to 30 minutes. Remove from the oven, season to taste with additional salt and black pepper, if needed and serve hot.

Kiwi Fruit

Native to China, the Kiwi fruit has a delicious sweet and tart flavor which most people love. They're an excellent source of fiber, vitamin C, vitamin K and vitamin B6, as well as several minerals and antioxidants – the skin contains the largest amount of antioxidants, unfortunately, since the fruit's fuzzy skin is simply discarded by many people.

Kiwi fruit is a natural fit for a fruit salad, smoothies or eaten out of hand as a snack or light breakfast. Try adding these unusual, yet delicious and very healthy fruits to your diet – you'll be glad that you did.

Kiwi Salsa

Number of servings: varies

Ingredients:

6 kiwis, peeled and diced
1 small sweet onion, diced
1 jalapeno pepper, diced
1 tbsp olive oil
1 tsp honey
½ tsp cumin
a pinch of chopped cilantro
juice of 2 limes
salt and black pepper, to taste

Preparation:

Mix together all of the ingredients in a bowl, except for the salt and pepper. Taste and season with salt and black pepper. Stir again, cover and allow the salsa to rest at room temperature for 1 hour. Refrigerate until ready to serve.

Spinach Salad with Kiwi and Strawberries

Number of servings: 6 – 8

Ingredients:

8 cups spinach, rinsed and torn into bite-size pieces
3 kiwis, peeled and sliced
8 strawberries, quartered
½ cup chopped walnuts
¼ cup canola oil
2 tbsp raspberry jam
2 tbsp raspberry vinegar

Preparation:

First, make your dressing by mixing together the vinegar, jam and oil in a small jar. Seal and shake vigorously to combine. Refrigerate until ready to use. In a large salad bowl, combine the remaining ingredients, then toss with the dressing and serve.

Kiwi Sandwiches

Number of servings: 8

Ingredients:

16 slices of whole grain bread
1 cup finely diced kiwi
1 cup cream cheese, softened at room temperature
zest of ½ lemon
2 tbsp honey

Preparation:

Mix the cream cheese, honey and lemon zest in a small bowl. Cover and refrigerate for 24 hours. Spread 2 tbsp of the cream cheese mixture on one slice of bread, then top with 2 tbsp of diced kiwi, then another slice of bread. Repeat this process to make all 8 sandwiches.

Kiwi Strawberry Smoothies

Number of servings: 2

Ingredients:

1 banana, halved
6 strawberries, quartered
1 kiwi, peeled and sliced
¾ cup pineapple juice
½ cup frozen yogurt

Preparation:

Place all of the ingredients in a blender and blend until smooth. Divide between 2 glasses and serve.

Fruit Pizza

Number of servings: varies (recipe makes 1 12" pizza)

Ingredients:

1 (18 ounce) package refrigerated sugar cookie dough
1 cup frozen whipped topping, thawed
1 banana, sliced
1 kiwi, sliced
½ cup sliced strawberries
½ cup crushed pineapple, drained

Preparation:

Preheat your oven to 350 F. Press the dough evenly into
a 12" pizza pan and bake until golden brown, 15 – 20
minutes. Remove from the oven and allow the crust to
cool to room temperature. Once the crust is cool, spread
it with the whipped topping and sliced fruit. Refrigerate
until ready to serve.

Blueberries

It's hard not to love blueberries. They have a taste which is uniquely their own and that almost everyone adores – but there's a lot more than taste to recommend these tart little berries. They're bursting with phytochemicals and antioxidants which are thought may help to combat cancer and other diseases and are also a source (albeit not a major source) of more than a dozen different vitamins and minerals.

Regular consumption of blueberries may also help to control cholesterol levels, reduce the risk of heart disease and possibly even help to improve memory. With all of these health benefits, it's no surprise that blueberries show up on any list of superfoods – and even if you aren't especially concerned about their nutritional value, their taste alone is enough to keep you coming back for more.

Blueberry Pie

Number of servings: varies (recipe makes 1 9" pie)

Ingredients:

4 cups fresh or frozen blueberries (thaw first if using frozen)
¾ cup sugar
2 tbsp corn starch
1 tbsp butter
½ tsp cinnamon
¼ tsp salt
1 9" inch double pie crust (premade or homemade)

Preparation:

Preheat your oven to 425 F. Mix together the corn starch, sugar, salt and cinnamon. Sprinkle this mixture over the blueberries. Line a 9" pie dish with one crust, pour in the blueberry mixture and dot the top with butter. Cut the other pie crust into ½" wide strips and make a lattice top. Crimp the edges with a fork. Bake for about 50 minutes, or until the crust of your pie is golden brown.

Blueberry Granita

Number of servings: 4

Ingredients:

2 ½ cups fresh blueberries
¾ cup water
½ cup sugar
juice of ½ lemon

Preparation:

Add the blueberries and sugar to a food processor and blend until smooth. Strain the mixture through a fine strainer, using a wooden spoon to press the mixture through while leaving as much of the seeds and skin behind as possible. Transfer the strained puree to a shallow glass tray and stir in the water and lemon juice. Place the tray in the freezer and freeze for about 4 hours, stirring once an hour. Scrape the granite from the tray and spoon into chilled small ice cream dishes for serving.

Blueberry Salsa

Number of servings: varies

Ingredients:

2 cups fresh blueberries, chopped roughly
1 cup fresh blueberries, whole
½ of a jalapeno pepper, minced (may use more or less to taste)
½ of a small red onion, diced
2 tbsp finely diced red bell pepper
juice of 2 limes
salt, to taste

Preparation:

Combine all of the ingredients in a bowl. Taste and season with salt, if desired. Cover and transfer to the refrigerator. Allow the salsa to chill for at least 2 hours before serving.

Blueberry Chicken

Number of servings: 4

Ingredients:

4 skinless, boneless chicken breast halves
2 cups fresh blueberries or frozen blueberries (thawed first)
½ cup white wine vinegar
2 tbsp Dijon mustard
2 tbsp orange marmalade
1 tbsp olive oil
salt and black pepper, to taste

Preparation:

Add the orange marmalade and Dijon mustard to a bowl. Stir well to combine. Heat oil over medium heat in a large, heavy skillet and cook the chicken for about 5 minutes per side, or until it's browned on the outside but still a little pink on the inside. Spread the marmalade and mustard mixture over the chicken add the blueberries and continue cooking until the chicken is completely cooked through, about 10 minutes, stirring frequently. The chicken is done when a meat thermometer inserted into the thickest part of a piece reads 165 F or higher. Transfer the cooked chicken to a serving plate.

Pour the vinegar into the skillet with the blueberries, season to taste with salt and black pepper. Cook until the sauce has been reduced by about 1/3. Pour the blueberry sauce over the chicken and serve.

Blueberry Walnut Salad

Number of servings: 6

Ingredients:

1 (10 ounce) package of mixed salad greens
2 cups fresh blueberries
½ cup raspberry vinaigrette (premade or homemade)
¼ cup roughly chopped walnuts
¼ cup crumbled feta cheese

Preparation:

Add the salad greens, walnuts, blueberries and salad dressing to a large bowl and toss to combine. Top the salad with crumbled feta and serve.

Dark Chocolate

Although chocolate isn't exactly a health food, at least in the form that we usually eat it, dark chocolate does have some health benefits which make it worthy of inclusion in this superfoods book. Cacao, the seeds which chocolate is made from, are rich in antioxidant compounds which prevent cell damage and inflammation – and these properties may make them useful in preventing certain cancers and other illnesses.

The healthiest way to eat chocolate is to have raw cacao, although this is generally too bitter for Western palates accustomed to chocolate which has been heavily sweetened. However, dark chocolate is the next best thing – you can still enjoy its health benefits by having it as an occasional treat instead of less healthy chocolate alternatives like milk and white chocolate.

Spicy Dark Chocolate Cookies

Number of servings: 36 cookies

Ingredients:

8 ounces semi-sweet chocolate, chopped
4 eggs
3 cups all-purpose flour
2 cups butter, softened at room temperature
2 cups brown sugar
1 ½ cups dark chocolate chips
1 cup white sugar
½ cup sifted cocoa powder
1 tbsp baking soda
1 tbsp water
1 tbsp vanilla extract
2 tsp minced chipotle peppers in adobo (may use more if you'd like spicier cookies)
1 tsp salt
a little powdered sugar, for coating the cookies before baking

Preparation:

Add the flour, salt and baking soda to a mixing bowl and

whisk together to combine. Set aside. Place the chocolate in a microwave safe bowl and melt; you can also use a double boiler to melt the chocolate, if you prefer. Let the chocolate cool a little bit before you proceed.

Beat the butter, brown and white sugar, chopped chipotle pepper and cocoa powder in a large bowl, mixing until the ingredients form a smooth mixture. Beat in the eggs one at a time. Add the water and vanilla extract to the mixture and stir well to combine. Next, add the melted chocolate, followed by the flour, salt and baking soda mixture and stir. Fold in the chocolate chips, then cover and place in the refrigerator for at least 1 hour to chill.

When you're ready to make the cookies, preheat your oven to 350 F and cover two large baking sheets with parchment paper. Roll small pieces of dough into balls, using your hands. You should end up with somewhere around three dozen cookies when all is said and done, but if you want to make larger cookies, feel free to do so.

Set the cookies on your parchment paper lined baking sheets, leaving at least 1" in between and preferably 2"; these cookies will spread out and flatten as they cook.

Bake for 12 – 15 minutes, remove from the oven and allow the cookies to cool for a few minutes, then transfer to wire racks to cool to room temperature. Store in an airtight sealed container.

Dark Chocolate Truffles

Number of servings: varies (recipe makes about 36 truffles)

Ingredients:

1 2/3 cups semi-sweet dark chocolate chips or finely chopped pieces
2/3 cups whipping cream (don't use light whipping cream for this recipe)
¼ cup finely chopped pistachios for coating the truffles.

Preparation:

Pour the whipping cream into a saucepan and bring to a boil, then immediately remove from heat. Add the chocolate chips or pieces and stir to melt the chocolate and incorporate both ingredients into a smooth mixture. Place the chocolate and whipping cream mixture in the refrigerator and allow it to cool and thicken for at least 15 minutes.

While the chocolate is cooling in the refrigerator, cover a baking sheet with parchment paper. Measure out a heaping teaspoon of the chocolate mixture for each truffle and place the baking sheet into the refrigerator to cool for another 20 minutes. Remove the truffles from the refrigerator, roll into balls by hand (you may want to lightly flour your hands to prevent excess sticking), then roll in the chopped pistachios to coat. Transfer the truffles into an airtight sealed container and refrigerate until you're ready to serve them.

Oats

Oats are a food that we should all be eating more of.
They're high in fiber and can help to regulate cholesterol
levels – and they're good for more than just porridge.
Oats can be included in soups, breads and all manner of
other foods; and they're so good for you that you just
might find yourself looking for excuses to include them
in other dishes once you've tried the oat recipes below.

Bannocks (Scottish Oat Cakes)

Number of servings: 2 – 4, depending on how large you
make them

Ingredients:

2 cups rolled oats
1 cup all purpose flour, sifted (you can also use ½ cup
whole wheat and ½ cup all purpose)
½ cup milk
½ cup butter, softened at room temperature
1 tbsp sugar
a pinch of salt
cooking spray

Start by preheating your oven to 375 F. Add the salt,
sugar, flour and baking powder to a sifter and sift well to
combine, into a large bowl. Add the oats and stir to mix,
then cut the butter into the dry ingredients using two
knives or a pastry cutter to form a pastry-like dough.
Add the milk a little bit at a time, stirring constantly.

Flour a work surface and turn out the dough. Roll out
the dough to about ½" thick. Divide the dough into two,
three or four pieces (depending how large you want to

make your bannocks), place on a baking sheet lightly coated with cooking spray and bake for about 15 minutes, or until the bannocks are lightly browned on top. Remove from the oven and serve warm or allow to cool to room temperature before serving.

Pumpkin

There's a lot more to pumpkins than Jack o' lanterns and pie (and actually, most canned pumpkin pie filling is made from butternut squash – all winter squash are pumpkins, technically speaking). Small pumpkins tend to be less watery and much easier to cook as well as sweeter, having a flavor very close to butternut or Hubbard squash.

Whether you use an actual orange pumpkin or another winter squash, these vegetables are excellent sources of vitamin A, beta carotene, vitamin C, omega-3 fatty acids, iron and B vitamins. Winter squash of all types are definitely superfoods in every sense of the word and as you'll see in these recipes, they're a perfect fit for dishes which are sweet, savory and everywhere in between.

New England Style Pumpkin Bread

Number of servings: varies (recipe yields 3 small loaves)

Ingredients:

3 cups all purpose flour
½ cup whole wheat flour
4 eggs
2 cups pureed pumpkin (canned or homemade)
2 cups white or turbinado sugar
1 cup canola oil
2/3 cup water
2 tsp baking soda
1 tsp salt
1 tsp each cinnamon, nutmeg and ground cloves
½ tsp powdered ginger

Preparation:

Start by preheating your oven to 350 F and prepare three small loaf pans by lightly greasing and then flouring them. Set aside. While your oven is preheating, add the eggs, oil, sugar, water and pumpkin to a large bowl and mix well to blend thoroughly.

Mix the rest of the dry ingredients in a bowl, whisking to combine. Add the dry ingredients to the wet ingredients and mix just until combined; pour the batter into your greased and floured loaf pans. Transfer the loaf pans to the oven and bake for about 50 minutes, or until a toothpick inserted into the center comes out clean.

Oatmeal with Pumpkin

Number of servings: 1

Ingredients:

½ cup rolled oats (or quick cooking oatmeal, if you want to save time)
1 cup milk or almond milk
¼ cup pureed pumpkin, canned or homemade
1 tsp honey, or more to taste
a pinch of cinnamon
a pinch of salt

Preparation:

Add all of the ingredients except for the honey to a small saucepan and bring to a boil, then reduce the heat to a simmer and cook until the oatmeal reaches your desired thickness, stirring regularly to prevent burning. Remove from heat, pour into a bowl and add 1 tsp honey or to taste.

Pumpkin Pasta

Number of servings: 6

Ingredients:

6 ounces uncooked very small pasta (your choice)
4 cups chicken or vegetable stock
1 medium sized yellow onion, diced
1 cup pumpkin, peeled, cubed and cooked (other winter
squash may be substituted if desired)
1 cup cooked turkey breast, cut into ½" pieces
2 tbsp olive oil or canola oil
1 tsp dried thyme
salt and black pepper, to taste
grated Romano cheese, for garnish

Preparation:

Pour the chicken or vegetable broth into a large
saucepan and bring to a slow boil over medium high
heat. In a large, heavy skillet, heat the olive oil over
medium heat. Saute the onion until tender, add the
thyme and then pour in about half of the stock
simmering in the saucepan.

Add the pasta to the skillet, stir and bring to a simmer. Add broth slowly, about half a cup at a time, stirring as you go and adding more once the broth is almost absorbed. Continue until the pasta is cooked to al dente texture, then add the butternut or acorn squash and cooked turkey. Stir well and add more broth, cooking until all of the ingredients are heated through, about 5 more minutes. Remove from heat, season to taste with salt and black pepper and serve hot garnished with a little grated Romano cheese.

Pumpkin Tacos or Tostadas

Number of servings: 12

Ingredients:

12 corn tortillas or tostada shells
2 cups of pumpkin, butternut squash or acorn squash
½ cup water
1 small red onion, diced
1 medium sized tomato, diced
2 tbsp canola oil or olive oil
1 tbsp cumin
1 tsp ancho chili powder
salt and black pepper, to taste
sliced avocado, chopped cilantro, salsa and lime wedges, for serving

Preparation:

Heat the canola or olive oil over medium heat in a large skillet or saucepan. Once the oil is hot, add the pumpkin or squash and cook for about 3 minutes, stirring occasionally. Add the stock and cumin, stir and continue cooking until the pumpkin or squash is fork tender, about 8 minutes. Season to taste with salt and black pepper, stir and divide the pumpkin mixture among the tortillas or tostada shells and serve topped with avocado slices and cilantro, with lime wedges and your choice of salsa on the side.

Superfoods Conclusion

You don't have to be a nutritionist to understand how much eating the superfoods featured in this book can benefit your health – and as you've already found out if you've been preparing these recipes, you don't have to be some kind of joyless health nut to enjoy eating them either!

Superfoods are all around us and you probably eat many of these foods already. Getting the most out of these foods is a matter of making a conscious decision to make them regular parts of your diet and of course, to try eating them raw when possible. Obviously, you're not going to want to eat raw quinoa, sweet potato or pumpkin, but don't overcook your food and you'll find that it tastes better as well as being healthier.

Eating superfoods should be part of a healthier lifestyle which includes a healthy diet and regular exercise. These healthy lifestyle habits work together to help you get the maximum nutrition that these foods offer and help you achieve better health and youthful energy which can last a lifetime.

Section 2: Dairy Free Diet

This Dairy Free Diet recipe book contains over 50 recipes that are 100% dairy free. Some of the recipes are ones you would not expect to find in a book like this like Mac and Cheese, cheesy casseroles, lasagna. There are also breakfast recipes that include muffins, breads, pancakes, and smoothies. You will find lunch recipes of sandwiches and soups and the supper section is the largest with a complete selection of dishes using vegetables, tuna, shrimp, beef, chicken and turkey, plus a few vegan dishes. All the recipes are delicious and fall in lines of a total dairy free diet.

Some of the dessert recipes include Apple Crumb Dessert, Fudge, Yellow Cake, Crunchy Oatmeal Cookies, Coconut Flavored Rice Pudding, Chocolate Pudding, Cheese Popcorn, Pumpkin Pie, Chocolate Rice Crispy Bars, and Banana Coconut Honey Oat Bars. Find recipes here that include cream soups like Cream of Chicken Soup, Potato Soup, and Split Pea Soup. You do not have to go without your favorite creamy foods. There is also a recipe for cream corn here!

Want to fix hearty foods to entertain a crowd? Try the

Rack of Lamb, Mango and Tuna Steaks, Honey Rolled Chicken Kabobs, or the Chicken and Dumplings. Want to please children? Try the Chicken Noodle Soup, Basic Fried Chicken, Mac and Cheese, Chicken A La King, "Cheesy" Vegetable Casserole, or the Turkey Burgers. Whatever flavor and style of cooking you like you will find a recipe here to suit your style and flavor. Also included are many family favorites and comfort foods.

Benefits of Dairy Free - Why People Choose Dairy Free

Eating dairy free helps to eliminate the junk foods from the diet. One of the biggest benefits to dairy free is the ability to lose unwanted fat and weight. Today more than ever there is support for engaging in such a diet plan, with many products at the market that are free of dairy ingredients. Eating a dairy free diet along with exercise and drinking plenty of water will help a person to shed the unwanted pounds and fat.

Some of the other benefits of going dairy free are the alleviation of certain physical conditions that tend to be aggravated by dairy foods otherwise. People express feeling less anxious and stressed when they rid dairy from their diets, not only is the stress gone but the energy levels rise. This enables an otherwise sedentary person the energy to get up and do physical activities, which further aids in weight loss. Another good benefit is the help in controlling the cholesterol and blood pressure levels.

Lactose intolerance is a big issue for many adults and the

presence of this condition merits going on a dairy free diet. You will find recipes that quickly substitute your favorite dishes less the milk and will be able to eat your favorite foods once again.

Adults are not the only ones who benefit from a dairy free diet children do too. Studies show children with conditions like autism and hyperactivity show improved behavior and reactions when the dairy foods are removed from their diet. Because many of the recipes here are delicious and fun to eat, children on these special diets will not be missing their favorite foods.

Improved health happens a lot while on a diary free diet being the main reason so many is trying it now. Removing dairy foods from the diet helps to control and sometimes even stop certain health conditions. If you have issues that are aggravated by eating milk products, it is worth a try to go a couple of weeks on a dairy free diet. Dairy foods are the cause of more food allergies than most other foods combined. Even moms who breast feed may pass on dairy products to their baby that may exhibit signs of dairy allergies. For those moms it would be wise to try dairy free foods until she weans her baby from breastfeeding. She may find she feels better too without the milk products.

The dairy free diet has other benefits like helping people to gain muscle mass as it helps to shed fat weight. Normally the benefits of such a diet take a little under two weeks to start seeing the benefits. This is enough time to develop a good habit of changing the diet plan.

How to Cope When You're a Dairy Lover, but For Health Reasons You Must Go Dairy Free

There are some good diary food substitutes out there to help ease into a dairy free diet. If you enjoy your glass of milk, or milk on your cereal, you can use milk made from almonds, hemp seeds, oats, rice, or soy. These versions of milk come in calcium fortified so you can pour it over your bowl of cereal or use in your recipes to know you are receiving the dietary calcium your body needs.

Cheese is another big issue for dairy lovers. Cheese substitutes do a nice job in helping to continue to eat the foods you love. Rice and soy both make cheese substitutes. Care must be made when choosing a cheese substitute and choose those without any dairy ingredients. Some imitation cheeses may contain casein, which is derived from milk as a milk protein. Another option for cheese is the varieties made from goat or sheep milk.

Butter lovers can find relief from dairy in the form of

margarine, which is butter-like spreads made from oils. Yogurts are made from rice and soy too and normally are found in health food stores. They come in plain and fruit. You can also create your own flavor with the plain rice or soy yogurts.

Dairy free ice cream does a great job at replacing the ice cream cravings. The same milk substitutes are made into delicious dairy-free ice creams. Other ice cream alternatives are sherbets because these are not made from milk products. If you have access to a good health food store you can find the milk substitute products including sour creams and all sorts of imitation cheeses.

Go ahead and make pizzas and ice cream, just use the dairy substitutes. Knowing the foods that sneak in dairy ingredients helps to remain dairy free too. Aside from the obvious milk, cheese, ice cream, yogurt, and butter avoid these foods: chocolate (read the ingredients), dips, whey powder, mayonnaise, coffee creamer (even the non-dairy contains casein milk protein), canned cream soups, cold cut lunch meats (look for turkey or chicken that contains no additives or preservatives).

These are ingredients that may sneak into foods, so watch out for: lactic acid, lactate, lactalbumin, lactoglobulin, casein, caseinate, galactose, acidophilus milk, ghee, curds, nougat, potassium caseinate, sodium caseinate, malted milk, rennet, and whey.

Eating out at restaurants can be a challenge when it comes to a dairy free diet. Avoid Mexican and Italian, which each contains dishes riddled with dairy foods. Choose Oriental foods instead. Vegan restaurants that are dairy free. If eating at a general restaurant choose meals made of grilled meats, steamed vegetables, fresh fruits and always ask for them to leave the butter and cheese off. A salad bar will allow control over the meal choosing a vinegar dressing.

Dairy free cookbooks such as this one will help to come up with recipes and ideas for foods to cook. If you are dairy free due to cow's milk issues, ask about trying goat or sheep milk and milk products too. Many regular grocers carry goat's milk and goat's milk cheeses.

Even Children Will Love These Recipes

Having a child with dairy allergies makes it difficult at times for them to have the foods they love. The recipes in this cookbook are ones kids will enjoy and some are even fun to make and eat. Included are recipes for different flavored pancakes, hot cocoa, mac and cheese, turkey burgers, and a whole section on desserts and snacks. Children will love the yellow cake, the chocolate pudding, the fudge, the crunchy oatmeal cookies and more.

Dairy Free Food List

In order to have a comprehensive list of true dairy free foods you need to read the ingredients on every package and refer to the list of diary-foods above for reference. Generally, the obvious foods are meats, vegetables, fruits, nuts, and grains. Any dairy-free milk substitute product made from rice or soy to substitute for milk, ice cream, and yogurt. Margarines made from oils.

Sample 5 Day Dairy Free Diet Plan

An asterisk* indicates the recipe is included in this book. The snacks are to be eaten between the meals and for dessert after supper. In addition to the "2" snacks listed, include nuts, raw vegetables and fruit mixed in with the foods. This is a sampling of meals using some of the recipes in this dairy free diet recipe book. Feel free to add extra vegetables and fruits to the meals.

Day 1-

Breakfast - Buckwheat Walnut Muffins*, eggs, sausage (turkey, soy or pork), juice.

Lunch - Pork Barbecue Sandwiches*, French fries, Coleslaw*, beverage (tea or water or juice)

Supper - Tuna Casserole*, salad with vinaigrette dressing, beverage (tea, water or juice)

Snacks - Apple Crumb Dessert*, Fudge*

Day 2-

Breakfast - Milk Free Latte*, Orange Banana Berry Pancakes*, bacon (turkey or soy)

Lunch - Chicken and Fruit Salad*, beverage (water, tea or juice)

Supper - Salisbury Steak*, Mac and Cheese*, baked potato with margarine, salad with vinaigrette dressing, beverage (tea, water or juice)

Snacks - Yellow Cake*, Crunchy Oatmeal Cookies*

Day 3-

Breakfast - Hot Cocoa*, Crepes*, bacon (turkey, soy or pork), orange slices

Lunch - Clam Chowder*, salad with vinaigrette dressing, beverage (water, tea or juice)

Supper - Chicken Tortilla Soup, salad with vinaigrette dressing, beverage (tea, water or juice)

Snacks - Coconut Flavored Rice Pudding*, Cheese Popcorn*

Day 4-

Breakfast - Banbergo Smoothie*, Basic Pancakes*, sausage (turkey, soy or pork)

Lunch - Chicken Noodle Soup*, salad with vinaigrette dressing, saltine crackers, beverage (water, tea or juice)

Supper - Beefy Cabbage Casserole*, beverage (tea, water or juice)

Snacks - Chocolate Pudding*, Banana Coconut Honey Oat Bars*

Day 5-

Breakfast - Breakfast Banana Smoothie*, Granola Bars*

Lunch - Super Easy Vegetable Beef Soup*, salad with vinaigrette dressing, saltine crackers, beverage (water, tea or juice)

Supper - Grilled Garlic Shrimp*, Coleslaw*, Cream Corn*, steamed vegetables, beverage (tea, water or juice)

Snacks - Pumpkin Pie*, Chocolate Rice Crispy Bars*

Kids Can Enjoy Dairy Free Diet Too

Thanks to soy, rice, and almond milk, kids will still get their yummy frozen treats. Make homemade dairy free ice creams, flavor it with fruits and nuts. Since there exists substitutes for all the dairy foods, kids will not have to feel like they are doing without their favorite meals. Make pizzas and cheeseburgers with cheese substitutes. Most recipes are okay if you substitute the milk ingredient with soy or rice milk. Just make sure to read through the recipe and see if they list any warnings about it.

Recipes:

Dairy Free Breakfast Recipes

Applesauce

Makes 4 servings

Ingredients:

*3 cups of apples (chopped, no peels and no core)
*3/4 cup of water
*1/4 cup of sugar (granulated)
*1/2 teaspoon of cinnamon (ground)

Directions:

Pour the 3 cups of apples into a saucepan turn heat to medium. Add the 2/3 cup of water, 1/4 cup of granulated sugar and 1/2 teaspoon of ground cinnamon. Place lid on pan and cook for about 20 minutes. Apples are done when they are soft, easily pierced with a fork.

Remove from heat and cool to room temperature. Place apples and liquid in a blender and blend until smooth. Or mash with a fork or a potato masher until the chunks are gone.

Buckwheat Walnut Muffins

Makes 8 servings.

Ingredients:

*3/4 cups of buckwheat flour
1 1/2 cups of apples (finely chopped or grated)
*1/4 cup of flax seeds (ground)
*1/2 cup of almond milk
*1/2 cup of walnuts (chopped)
*1 egg
*3 tablespoons of coconut oil
*2 tablespoons of dairy free margarine
*1 tablespoon of honey
*1 teaspoon of baking powder
*1 teaspoon of cinnamon (ground)
*1/4 teaspoon of salt

Directions:

Preheat oven to 350 degrees Fahrenheit. Grease 8 cups in a dozen cup muffin pan.

In a large bowl add the 3/4 cup of buckwheat flour, 1/4 cup of ground flax seeds, 1 teaspoon of baking powder,

1 teaspoon of ground cinnamon and 1/4 teaspoon of salt and mix. In a different bowl add the egg and beat. Stir in the 1 1/2 cups of grated apples, 1/2 cup of almond milk, and 3 tablespoons of coconut oil. Do not over stir. Mix in the dry ingredients, careful not to over stir again. Fold in the 1/2 cup of walnuts. Spoon the batter evenly into the 8 cups and bake for 25 minutes until golden brown. Muffins are done with inserted toothpick in the middle comes out clean. Mix softened 2 tablespoons of margarine with the 1 tablespoon of honey and spread over the top of the muffins.

Pumpkin Spice Muffins

Makes 10 servings.

Ingredients:

*2 cups of whole wheat flour
*1 can of pumpkin (15 oz)
*1/2 cup of sugar (granulated)
*1/2 cup of raisins
*1/2 cup of water
*1 tablespoon of baking powder
*1/2 teaspoon of baking soda
*1/2 teaspoon of salt
*1/2 teaspoon of cinnamon (ground)
*1/4 teaspoon of nutmeg (ground)

Directions:

Preheat oven to 375 degrees. Spray 10 muffin cups with cooking spray and set aside. In a bowl mix the 2 cups of flour with the 1/2 cup of granulated sugar, 1 tablespoon of baking powder, 1/2 teaspoon of baking soda, 1/2 teaspoon of salt, 1/2 teaspoon of ground cinnamon, and the 1/4 teaspoon of ground nutmeg. Stir in the can of pumpkin, 1/2 cup of water, and the 1/2 cup of raisins.

Spoon into the 10 muffin cups. Bake for half an hour or until the tops turn golden brown and are springy. Cool for 5 minutes, then serve warm.

Milk Free Latte

Makes 2 servings.

Ingredients:

*1 1/4 cups of rice milk (plain)
*3 teaspoons of instant coffee
*2 teaspoons of sugar (granulated)

Add the 1 1/4 cups of rice milk, 3 teaspoons of instant coffee, and 2 teaspoons of granulated sugar in a saucepan and turn heat to medium. Stir constantly and remove when liquid steams. Pour into 2 cups and enjoy.

Banana Nut Bread

Makes 6 to 8 servings.

Ingredients:

*1 1/2 cup of flour (all-purpose)
*1 cup of sugar (granulated)
*1/2 cup of canola oil
*1/4 cup of walnuts (finely chopped)
*3 bananas (ripe and mashed)
*1 egg
*1 teaspoon of baking soda
*1/4 teaspoon of salt

Directions:

Preheat oven to 325 degrees Fahrenheit. Spray loaf pan with oil/flour cooking spray. In a bowl, mix the 1 cup of sugar with the 1/2 cup of canola oil. Beat the egg first, and then stir in the batter. Add the 1 1/2 cups of all-purpose flour, 1 teaspoon of baking soda and 1 teaspoon of salt. Fold in the 3 mashed bananas and the 1/4 cup of finely chopped walnuts. Pour batter into the greased loaf pan and bake until toothpick inserted in the middle comes out clean, for about 60 minutes.

Basic Pancakes

Makes 6 servings.

Ingredients:

*2 cups of water
*1 cup of rice flour
*1/3 cup of potato starch
*2 eggs
*3 tablespoons of tapioca flour
*3 tablespoons of canola oil
*1 tablespoon of brown sugar
*1 1/2 teaspoons of baking powder
*1/2 teaspoon of baking soda
*1/2 teaspoon of salt
*1/2 teaspoon of guar gum
*margarine
*syrup

Directions:

Mix the 1 cup of rice flour, 1/3 cup of potato starch, 3 tablespoons of tapioca flour, 1 tablespoon of brown sugar, 1 1/2 teaspoons of baking powder, 1/2 teaspoon of baking soda, 1/2 teaspoon of salt and the 1/2 teaspoon of guar gum together in a bowl. Beat the 2 eggs and stir into the dry ingredients along with the 2 cups of water and 3 tablespoons of canola oil. Spray with cooking spray a griddle or a flat skillet or pan and warm to medium high heat. Spoon about 1/4 cup of batter onto the hot griddle or pan and cook until the middle bubbles and the bottom turns a golden brown, about 4 minutes. Carefully flip and cook until golden brown, 2 to 3 minutes. Add a pat of margarine and drizzle with syrup, serve immediately.

Orange Banana Berry Pancakes

Makes 4 servings.

Ingredients:

*1 cup of oat flour
*1 cup of rice milk
*1 cup of blueberries
*3/4 cup of orange juice (pulp free is best)
*2/3 cup of whole wheat flour
*10 strawberries (mashed)
*1 banana (mashed)
*1 tablespoon of baking powder
*1 tablespoon of sugar (granulated)
*1/4 teaspoon of salt

Directions:

In a bowl mix the 1 cup of oat flour, 2/3 cup of whole wheat flour, 1 tablespoon of baking powder, 1 tablespoon of granulated sugar and 1/4 teaspoon of salt and set aside. In a separate bowl, mix the strawberries and banana together until smooth. Fold in the 1 cup of blueberries and then add the 1 cup of rice milk, and the 3/4 cup of pulp free orange juice, stir until blended.

Gently fold the dry ingredients into the fruit batter, stirring until blended. If the batter is too thick, add a little more rice milk. Allow the batter to sit for a few minutes while preheating the griddle or a flat pan to around 350 degrees Fahrenheit or medium high. If needed lightly spray the pan or griddle with cooking spray. Pour about 1/4 cup of batter onto the hot pan or griddle. Cook until the bottom begins to brown, the top will produce bubbles, takes about 5 minutes. Flip over and cook until bottom is golden brown, about 3 minutes. Add a pat of margarine and serve immediately with pancake syrup.

Breaded Pancakes

Makes 8 servings.

Ingredients:

*3/4 cup of breadcrumbs
*3/4 cup of soymilk
*1/4 cup of whole wheat flour
*2 eggs
*1 tablespoon of canola oil
*2 teaspoons of baking powder
*1/4 teaspoon of salt

Directions:

Put the 3/4 cup of breadcrumbs in a bowl and cover with the 3/4 cup of soymilk and the 1 tablespoon of canola oil. Meanwhile in a separate bowl mix the 1/4 cup of flour, 2 teaspoons of baking powder and 1/4 teaspoon of salt together. Beat the 2 eggs and add to the flour mixture. Stir in the breadcrumbs and milk. Spoon 1/4 cup of breadcrumb batter onto a hot griddle or skillet that was sprayed with cooking spray. Cook until bottom is golden brown, flip and cook until bottom is golden brown. Serve immediately.

NOTE: Good served with a pat of margarine and a sprinkling of powdered sugar or a drizzle of maple-flavored syrup.

Crepes

Makes 4 servings.

Ingredients:

*1 cup of rice flour
*1/2 cup of coconut milk
*1/4 cup of water
*2 tablespoons of cornstarch
*1/2 teaspoon of sugar (granulated)
*1/2 teaspoon of salt

Directions:

Add the 1 cup of rice flour, 2 tablespoons of cornstarch, 1/2 teaspoon of granulated sugar, and 1/2 teaspoon of salt to a bowl and stir. Add in the 1/2 cup of coconut milk and the 1/4 cup of water and stir. Heat a griddle or large skillet sprayed with cooking spray to medium high heat. Spoon 1/4 cup of the crepe batter onto the hot pan and cook until the edges start to brown and curl. Flip and cook until golden brown. Serve with favorite syrup or fruits.

Hot Cocoa

Makes 4 servings.

Ingredients:

*4 cups of soymilk
*8 tablespoons of sugar (granulated)
*3 tablespoons of cocoa (unsweetened powder)
*1 teaspoon of vanilla extract

Directions:

In a large saucepan, add the 4 cups of soymilk and turn heat to medium high. Stir in the 8 tablespoons of granulated sugar and 3 tablespoons of unsweetened cocoa powder, and 1 teaspoon of vanilla extract. Stir constantly until the cocoa becomes steamy. Serve immediately in mugs.

NOTE: For an added treat, add a peppermint stick in each mug.

Granola Bars

Makes 16 servings.

Ingredients:

*1 3/4 cups of oats (rolled)
*1 cup of crisp rice cereal
*3/4 cup of brown sugar
*3/4 cup of rice flour
*1/2 cup of walnuts or peanuts or almonds (chopped)
*1/2 cup of semisweet chocolate chips
*1/3 cup of margarine (softened)
*2 tablespoons of honey
*1 egg
*1 teaspoon of guar gum
*1 teaspoon of vanilla extract
*1 teaspoon of baking soda
*1/4 teaspoon of salt

Directions:

Preheat the oven to 350 degrees Fahrenheit. Spray a 9x13 pan with cooking spray. Add the 3/4 cup of brown sugar in a bowl with the 1/3 cup of margarine, cream together. Beat the egg, add to the batter, and stir in the

2 tablespoons of honey and 1 teaspoon of vanilla extract. Mix until creamy smooth. In a separate bowl add the 3/4 cup of rice flour, 1 teaspoon of guar gum, 1 teaspoon of baking soda and 1/4 teaspoon of salt. Gradually add to the batter, stirring well. Fold in the 1 3/4 cups of rolled oats, 1 cup of crisp rice cereal, 1/2 cup of chopped nuts, and 1/2 cup of semisweet chocolate chips. Spoon the mixture into the sprayed 9x13 pan. Pat down and bake until golden brown, about 20 minutes. Cool and cut into squares and serve.

Banbergo Smoothie

Makes 6 servings.

Ingredients:

*2 bananas (ripe, peeled, chopped and frozen)
*2 mangoes (frozen, peeled and chopped)
*2 cup of orange juice
*2 cups of strawberries (chopped)
*2 tablespoons of honey
*1 tablespoon of lemon juice

Directions:

Add the 2 cups of chopped strawberries to a blender and blend. Add in the 2 chopped frozen bananas and the 2 frozen chopped mangoes and "chop and blend" in the blender until smooth. Add in the 2 cups of orange juice, 2 tablespoons of honey and 1 tablespoon of lemon juice and blend for a couple of minutes until the texture is nice and smooth. Pour into 6 glasses and serve immediately.

Banana Blueberry Smoothie

Makes 4 servings.

Ingredients:

*4 cups of soymilk
*3 cups of blueberries
*4 ripe bananas
*1/2 cup of soy protein powder
*4 tablespoons of flax seed meal

Directions:

Put the 4 cups of soymilk and 3 cups of blueberries in a blender followed by the 4 ripe bananas (cut them into large chunks), 1/2 cup of soy protein powder and 4 tablespoons of flax seed meal. Blend until all ingredients are smooth. Serve immediately. If you wish, you may add a drizzle of honey to the mixture for extra sweetness.

Breakfast Banana Smoothie

Makes 4 servings.

Ingredients:

*2 ripe bananas
*3 cups of water
*1 cups of ice

Directions:

Add the bananas along with 3 cups of water and 1 cup of ice to a blender. Blend until smooth. Serve immediately.

Make a strawberry banana smoothie by adding a few ripe strawberries. Sweeten with honey if desired.

Lunch and Supper Recipes

Pork (or Lamb) Barbecue Sandwiches

Makes 6 servings.

*1 1/2 pounds of pork (or better -- lamb) ribs (deboned)
*1 1/8 cups of barbecue sauce
*1 cup of beef broth

Directions:

Add the 1 1/2 pounds of boneless pork ribs and the 1 cup of beef broth into a Crockpot. Cook for 3 to 4 hours on high, until meat is tender and easily shreds with a fork. Shred pork with forks. Place the shredded pork into a baking dish and cover with the 1 1/8 cups of barbecue sauce and cook in 350 degrees Fahrenheit oven for half an hour.

Serve on dairy-free buns or bread.

Chicken and Fruit Salad

Makes 6 servings.

Ingredients:

*1 pound of chicken breasts (skinless and boneless)
*2 heads of iceberg lettuce (washed, dried and torn into bite sized pieces)
*1 cup of strawberries
*1 cup of canola oil
*1/2 cup of pecans
*1/2 cup of sugar (granulated)
*1/3 cup of red wine vinegar
*1/2 onion (minced)
*1 teaspoon of mustard (ground)
*1 teaspoon of salt
*1/4 teaspoon of black pepper

Directions:

Prepare the grill for cooking the chicken. If no grill cook on the top rack of the oven under the broiler with a cookie sheet underneath to catch the drippings. Spray the grill with cooking spray, or lightly spray the chicken if cooking in the oven under the broiler. Cook about 7 or 8 minutes, making sure it is cooked to the center and the juices are running clear. Remove from grill or boiler and let cool a few minutes. Slice into strips. Heat a dry skillet to medium high heat and add the pecans for about 8 minutes, stirring often, and turning. Take off heat and place in bowl. Add the 1 cup of canola oil, 1/2 cup of granulated sugar, 1/3 cup of red wine vinegar, 1/2 minced onion, 1 teaspoon of ground mustard, 1 teaspoon of salt and 1/4 teaspoon of black pepper to a blender and blend until smooth. Divide the lettuce among 6 plates; divide the grilled chicken strips on top of the lettuce, as well as the cup of strawberries and half cup of toasted pecans. Pour the dressing over the top and serve immediately.

Clam Chowder

Makes 6 servings.

Ingredients:

*4 cups of potatoes (peeled and diced - russet or baking)
*3 cups of rice milk
*2 cups of clam broth
*2 cans of minced clams (6.5 oz)
*2 carrots (peeled and sliced)
*1 onion (diced)
*1 bay leaf
*1/2 cup of flour (all purpose)
*1 tablespoon olive oil
*1 tablespoon of parsley (dried)
*3/4 teaspoon of salt
*1/2 teaspoon of thyme (crushed)
*1/2 teaspoon of white pepper
*1/4 teaspoon of black pepper (ground)
*salt and pepper to season
*saltine crackers

Directions:

Pour the tablespoon of oil into a stockpot and heat on

medium heat. Stir in the diced onion and the 2 sliced carrots. Stir and sauté until vegetables are soft. Add the flour, stirring for the roux, bust the clumps. Gradually add the 2 cups of clam broth, stirring until smooth. Stir in the 3 cups of rice milk. Add the 2 cans of minced clams along with the bay leaf, 1 tablespoon of dried parsley, 3/4 teaspoon of salt, 1/2 teaspoon crushed thyme, 1/2 teaspoon white pepper, and the 1/4 teaspoon of ground black pepper. Turn the temperature to high and bring to a boil while stirring often. Turn the heat down to simmer, put a lid on the pot, and simmer for half an hour. Add the 4 cups of diced potatoes and simmer another half an hour until soft. Remove bay leaf. Season with salt and pepper and serve with saltine crackers.

Chicken Noodle Soup

Makes 6 servings.

Ingredients:

*2 pounds of chicken (skinned, deboned and chopped)
*8 cups of water
*2 stalks of celery (chopped)
*1 onion (chopped)
*1 carrot (peeled and finely chopped)
*1 bay leaf
*6 ounces of noodles (flat egg noodles work well)
*1/4 cup of parsley (fresh chopped)
*1 tablespoon of salt
*1 teaspoon of seasoning (Mrs. Dash, Accent, or similar)
*1/2 teaspoon of basil
*1/4 teaspoon of black pepper (ground)

Directions:

Add the 8 cups of water to the Crockpot turned to high temperature and add the 2 pounds of chopped chicken, 2 chopped stalks of celery, 1 chopped onion, 1 peeled and finely chopped carrot, 1/4 cup of fresh chopped parsley, bay leaf, 1 tablespoon of salt, 1 teaspoon of seasoning, 1/2 teaspoon basil, and 1/4 teaspoon of ground black pepper. Cook for 5 hours and 30 minutes. Remove the bay leaf and add the 6 ounces of noodles and cook for 30 minutes. Add to soup tureen and cool slightly before serving.

Super Easy Vegetable Beef Soup

Makes 6 servings.

Ingredients:

*1 pound of ground beef
*1 can of tomatoes (28 oz - chopped)
*2 cans of beef broth (10.5 oz)
*1 can of green beans (16 oz)
*3 cups of potatoes (diced)
*2 cups of water
*1 cup of celery (chopped)
*1 cup of carrots (sliced)
*1 cup of onions (chopped)
*2 teaspoons of chili powder
*3 dashes of cayenne pepper sauce
*1 teaspoon of salt
*1 teaspoon of Worcestershire sauce

Directions:

Cook the pound of ground beef in a skillet, drain the fat and put the beef in a Crockpot. Add all the remaining ingredients and stir. Turn Crockpot to high for an hour, then on low for another 7 hours. Allow to cool slightly before serving.

NOTE: Add a few noodles during the last hour of cooking if desired. Add other vegetables like leftovers from the previous week too.

Cream of Chicken Soup

Makes 4 servings.

Ingredients:

*2 cups of chicken broth
*1/2 cup of chicken (cooked, finely chopped)
*2 potatoes (peeled and diced)
*1 carrot (peeled and thinly sliced)
*1/2 cup of celery (chopped)
*1/4 cup of celery leaves
*salt and pepper to season

Directions:

Pour the 2 cups of chicken broth into a pot and bring to a boil. Stir in the 2 diced potatoes, sliced carrot and the 1/2 cup of chopped celery with the 1/4 cup of celery leaves, bring to another boil. Put lid on pot and turn heat to simmer for 25 minutes. Allow to cool slightly, pour entire pot into a blender, and blend until smooth. Return to pot and add the 1/3 cup of cooked chicken and heat through. Serve warm.

Potato Soup

Makes 6 servings.

Ingredients:

*8 potatoes (peeled and diced)
*2 cups of chicken broth
*2 2/3 cups of water
*1 onion (chopped)
*7 slices of bacon (chopped)
*2/3 cup of bell pepper (chopped)
*2/3 cup of cheddar cheese substitute
*2/3 cup of rice milk
*4 tablespoons of green onions (finely sliced)
*2 tablespoons of margarine
*salt and pepper to season.

Add all ingredients to a Crockpot and cook on high for 4
hours or until the potatoes are softened. If desired,
mash the potatoes with a potato masher. Season with
salt and pepper.

Split Pea Soup

Makes 6 servings.

Ingredients:

*6 cups of chicken or vegetable broth
*1 package of split peas (16 oz. dried and rinsed)
*2 cups of ham (diced)
*1 1/2 cups of carrots (thinly sliced)
*1/2 cup of onions (chopped)
*2 stalks of celery (chopped with leaves)
*2 cloves of garlic (minced)
*1 bay leaf
*1/2 tablespoon of seasoning salt
*1/2 teaspoon of black pepper (ground)

Directions:

Pour the package of split peas into the bottom of a Crockpot. On top of that place the 2 cups of ham, 1 1/2 cups of thinly sliced carrots, 1/2 cup of chopped onion, 2 chopped stalks of celery and leaves and the bay leaf. Sprinkle on top of that the 1/2 tablespoon of seasoning salt and the 1/2 teaspoon of ground black pepper. Pour the 6 cups of broth over the top, no need to stir. Cook on high for 4 and a half hours, or until the peas are tender. OR cook over night on low for a total of at least 8 hours. Remove the bay leaf. Transfer to a soup tureen or large serving bowl to cool a little before serving.

Grilled Garlic Shrimp

Makes 6 servings.

Ingredients:

*2 pounds of shrimp (peeled and deveined)
*3 garlic cloves (minced)
*1/3 cup of olive oil
*1/4 cup of tomato sauce
*2 tablespoons of red wine vinegar
*2 tablespoons of basil (fresh chopped)
*1/2 teaspoon of salt
*1/4 teaspoon of cayenne pepper

Directions:

Add to a bowl the 3 minced garlic cloves, 1/3 cup of olive oil, 1/4 cup of tomato sauce and the 2 tablespoons of red wine vinegar and stir. Add the 2 tablespoons of fresh chopped basil, 1/2 teaspoon of salt and 1/4 teaspoon of cayenne pepper and stir. Add the 2 pounds of peeled deveined shrimp, tossing to coat. Cover the bowl and refrigerate for 45 minutes, tossing the shrimp every 15 minutes. Slightly oil a grill and heat to medium. Skewer the shrimp and cook for 3 minutes, then turn over and cook another 3 minutes. Do not reuse the marinade simply throw it away. Serve hot shrimp immediately.

Beefy Cabbage Casserole

Makes 6 servings.

Ingredients:

*1 1/2 pounds of lean ground beef
*1 cabbage (small size, shredded)
*1 can of tomato sauce (14 oz)
*1 cup of onions (finely chopped)
*1 cup of water
*1/2 cup of rice
*1 clove of garlic (minced)
*1 teaspoon of salt
*1/4 teaspoon of black pepper (ground)

Directions:

Brown the 1 1/2 pounds of lean ground beef in a skillet. Add the can of tomato sauce, 1 cup of finely chopped onions, 1 cup of water, 1 minced garlic clove, 1 teaspoon of salt and 1/4 teaspoon of ground black pepper and stir. Stir in the 1/2 cup of rice. Put a lid on and simmer until the rice is tender, about 20 minutes. Meanwhile preheat the oven to 350 degrees Fahrenheit. Spray a medium sized baking dish with cooking spray. Place half of the shredded cabbage on the bottom, cover with half of the beef mixture, add the remaining shredded cabbage and the remaining beef mixture. Cover with foil and bake for 60 minutes. All to cool for 10 minutes before serving.

Rack of Lamb

Makes 4 servings.

Ingredients:

*1 rack of lamb (7 bone trimmed)
*1/2 cup of bread crumbs (use fresh)
*2 tablespoons of garlic (minced)
*2 tablespoons of rosemary (fresh chopped)
*4 tablespoons of olive oil (divided)
*1 tablespoon of Dijon mustard
*2 teaspoons of salt (divided)
*1 1/4 teaspoon of black pepper (ground - divided)

Directions:

Preheat the oven to 450 degrees Fahrenheit. Pour the 1/2 cup of fresh bread crumbs into a bowl and toss in the 2 tablespoons of minced garlic cloves, 2 tablespoons of fresh chopped rosemary, 1 teaspoon of salt, and 1/4 teaspoon of ground black pepper. Drizzle 2 tablespoons of olive oil over the top and toss once more. Rub the remaining 1 teaspoon of salt and the teaspoon of ground black pepper on the rack of lamb. Heat the remaining 2 tablespoons of oil in a large skillet and brown the lamb, turning to all sides at least 2 minutes per side. Allow rack of lamb to cool for a couple of minutes, then rub the tablespoon of Dijon mustard over the lamb and then roll the rack of lamb in the bread crumbs, coating all sides evenly. Place foil on the ends of each bone. Place the rack of lamb in a baking dish or the skillet and place in oven for 18 minutes to well done. Remove from oven and allow cooling for about 6 minutes. Carve and serve.

Tuna Casserole

Makes 6 servings.

Ingredients:

*3 1/2 cups of brown rice pasta
*2 cans of tuna (6 oz packed in water)
*2 cups of chicken broth
*1 cup of mushrooms (sliced)
*3/4 cup of bread crumbs
*1/2 cup of peas (frozen)
*1/2 cup of onions (chopped)
*1/4 cup of olive oil mayonnaise
*1/4 cup of rice flour
*4 1/2 tablespoons of olive oil (divided)
*salt and pepper to season
*paprika to season

Directions:

Preheat the oven to 350 degrees Fahrenheit. Spray a
9x13 pan with cooking spray. In a skillet, add the 2
tablespoons of olive oil and heat to medium. Stir in the 1
cup of sliced mushrooms and 1/2 cup of chopped onions
and sauté. Put onions and mushrooms in a bowl. Drizzle

another 2 tablespoons of olive oil into the pan, heat up, and add the 1/4 cup of flour to make a roux, stirring with a whisk. Pour in the broth slowly, stirring constantly until it thickens into a bubbly gravy. Mix the 1/4 cup of olive oil mayonnaise and the salt and pepper in a cup, and then add the mixture to the gravy and stir. Drain the 2 cans of tuna and add to the gravy mixture along with the mushroom and onion mixture. Stir in the frozen peas. Place the 3 1/1 cups of brown rice pasta in the bottom of the baking dish, spreading evenly. Pour the gravy sauce over the pasta. Sprinkle the 3/4 cup of breadcrumbs over the top. Sprinkle the paprika over the breadcrumbs and then drizzle the remaining 1/2 tablespoon of olive oil over that. Bake until the top turns a golden brown, about half an hour.

Mango and Tuna Steaks

Makes 4 servings.

Ingredients:

*4 tuna steaks
* 1 mango (peeled, pitted, chopped)
*1 jalapeno pepper (seeded, minced)
*2 garlic cloves (minced)
*1 green onion (chopped)
*1/4 cup of red bell pepper (finely chopped)
*1/4 cup of onion (finely chopped)
*6 tablespoons and 1 1/2 teaspoons of olive oil (divided)
*4 tablespoons of lime juice (divided)
*2 tablespoons of paprika
*2 tablespoons of cilantro (fresh chopped)
*1 tablespoon of cayenne pepper
*1 tablespoon of onion powder
*1 tablespoon of garlic powder
*2 teaspoons of salt
*1 teaspoon of black pepper (ground)
*1 teaspoon of thyme (dried)
*1 teaspoon of basil (dried)
*1 teaspoon of oregano (dried)

Directions:

In a small bowl add the 2 tablespoons of olive oil with the 2 tablespoons of lime juice and the 2 cloves of minced garlic, whisking together and then put on the 4 tuna steaks, rubbing into the entire steaks. Wrap the tuna steaks tightly and refrigerate for several hours. In a separate bowl add the chopped mango with the minced jalapeno pepper, chopped green onion, 1/4 cup of finely chopped red bell pepper, 1/4 cup of finely chopped onion and the 2 tablespoons of fresh chopped cilantro. Pour the 2 tablespoons of lime juice along with 1 1/2 teaspoons of olive oil over and toss for even coating. Cover and refrigerate for an hour. In a large plate mix the 2 tablespoons of paprika with the 1 tablespoon of cayenne pepper, tablespoon of garlic powder, tablespoon of onion powder, 2 teaspoons of salt, teaspoon of ground black pepper, teaspoon of dried thyme, teaspoon of dried basil and the teaspoon of dried oregano. After the tuna steaks have been refrigerated for at least 3 hours, rinse them with water, and drag through the spices, both sides with all 4 steaks. Add 2 tablespoons of olive oil in a large skillet and turn to medium heat. Cook the tuna steaks for 3 minutes then add the remaining olive oil and cook the other side of the tuna steaks for 3 minutes. Divide the mango salsa among 4 plates, place a tuna steak on top of the mangos, and serve while still hot.

Chicken Tortilla Soup

Makes 8 servings.

Ingredients:

*1 pound of chicken (cooked, shredded)
*tortilla chips (normal sized bag)
*1 can of tomatoes (15 oz, peeled and mashed)
*1 can of chicken broth (14.5 oz)
*1 can of enchilada sauce (10 oz)
*1 package of corn (10 oz frozen)
*1 can of green chili peppers (4 oz)
*2 cups of water
*1 bay leaf
*2 garlic cloves (minced)
*1 tablespoon of cilantro (chopped)
*1 teaspoon of cumin
*1 teaspoon of chili powder
*1 teaspoon of salt
*1/4 teaspoon of black pepper (ground)

Directions:

Turn Crockpot to high setting; add the pound of cooked shredded chicken and pour in the can of tomatoes, can of chicken broth, can of enchilada sauce and stir. Add the package of frozen corn, can of green chili peppers (liquid and all), 2 cups of water, 2 minced garlic cloves, tablespoon of chopped cilantro, teaspoon of cumin, teaspoon of chili powder, teaspoon of salt and 1/4 teaspoon of ground black pepper and stir. Cook for 3 1/2 hours. Serve in bowls and crumble tortilla chips over the top.

Salisbury Steak

Makes 6 servings.

Ingredients:

*1 1/2 pounds of lean ground beef
*1 can of French onion soup (condensed 10.5 oz)
*1/2 cup of bread crumbs
*1/4 cup of ketchup
*1/4 cup of water
*1 egg
*1 tablespoon of Worcestershire sauce
*1 tablespoon of flour (all-purpose)
*1/2 teaspoon of mustard powder
*1/4 teaspoon of salt
*1/8 teaspoon of black pepper (ground)

Directions:

Put the 1 1/2 pounds of raw ground beef in a bowl and to it a third of the can of condensed French onion soup, the egg (slightly beaten), 1/2 cup of breadcrumbs, 1/4 teaspoon of salt, and 1/8 teaspoon of pepper. With bare hands (or gloved) squish together, and then create six patties. Place the patties in a skillet heated to medium high heat and cook until both sides are brown, about 5 or 6 minutes each side. Drain the fat from the skillet turn heat to medium low. In a bowl, add the tablespoon of all-purpose flour and the remaining 2/3 can of French onion soup. Whisk until smooth. Add the 1/4 cup of ketchup, tablespoon of Worcestershire sauce and 1/2 teaspoon of mustard powder and stir. Drizzle over the Salisbury steaks, put a lid on, and cook for about 20 minutes, stirring often.

Balsamic Vinegar Chicken

Makes 6 servings.

Ingredients:

*6 chicken breast halves (boneless and skinless)
*1 can of tomatoes (14.5 oz diced)
*1 cup of onion (sliced thin)
*1/2 cup of balsamic vinegar
*2 tablespoons of olive oil
*1 teaspoon of basil (dried)
*1 teaspoon of oregano (dried)
*1 teaspoon of rosemary (dried)
*1 teaspoon of garlic salt
*1/2 teaspoon of thyme (dried)
*black pepper to season

Directions:

Rub the teaspoon of garlic salt on the chicken breasts, sprinkle with black pepper. Add the 2 tablespoons of olive oil to a skillet and heat to medium. Add the rubbed chicken breasts and the cup of thinly sliced onions, sauté the onions. Add the can of tomatoes along with the 1/2 cup of balsamic vinegar over the chicken. Stir in the teaspoons of dried basil, dried oregano, dried rosemary, and dried thyme. Turn the heat to medium low and simmer the chicken until it is well done, when the juices are clear, about 15 to 20 minutes. Serve immediately.

Honey Rolled Chicken Kabobs

Makes 12 servings.

Ingredients:

*8 chicken breasts halves (boneless, skinless cut into bite sized chunks)
*2 1/2 cups of onions (cut into bite-sized chunks)
*2 red bell peppers (cut into bite sized chunks)
*1/3 cup of honey
*1/3 cup of soy sauce
*1/4 cup of canola oil
*2 garlic cloves (minced)
*1/4 teaspoon of black pepper (ground)

Directions:

Add the 1/3 cup of honey, 1/3 cup of soy sauce, 1/4 teaspoon of ground black pepper and 1/4 cup of olive oil in a large bowl, stirring. Dip out a ladle full and reserve in a cup for later use. Place the chicken into the marinade and put the 2 1/2 cups of cut up onions, 2 cut up red bell peppers on top, cover the bowl and refrigerate for 2 hours. (Overnight marinade soak is okay too.) Oil the grill and heat on high. Skewer the chicken, onions, and peppers. Brush with the reserved ladle of marinade during cooking.

Cook for 15 minutes on each side on the grill. Serve immediately.

Basic Fried Chicken

Makes 6 servings.

Ingredients:

*6 chicken breast halves (boneless, skinless)
*2 cups of canola oil
*1 cup of saltine crackers (finely crumbled)
*1 egg
*2 tablespoons of flour (all-purpose)
*2 tablespoons of potato flakes (from instant potatoes)
*1 teaspoon of seasoned salt
*1/2 teaspoon of black pepper (ground)

Directions:

Mix the cup of saltine cracker crumbs with the 2
tablespoons of all-purpose flour, 2 tablespoons of
instant potato flakes, teaspoon of seasoned salt and 1/2
teaspoon of ground black pepper in a bowl. Beat the egg
in another bowl. Heat the 2 cups of canola oil in a deep
skillet or a deep-fryer on medium high heat or 350
degrees Fahrenheit. Drag the chicken breasts through
the beaten egg, then coat with the cracker crumb
coating by placing the crumb mixture in a gallon sized

zipper bag and adding the chicken breasts, one at a time and shaking until well coated. Fry in the deep oil until well done, when the coating turns golden brown and the juices from the chicken runs clear. Serve immediately, can be store in the refrigerator and eaten cold too.

Coleslaw

Makes 8 servings.

Ingredients:

*1/2 cabbage (shredded)
*1 cup of carrots (shredded)
*4 tablespoons of raisins
*4 tablespoons of peanuts (toasted and salted)
*2 tablespoons of white wine vinegar
*2 tablespoons of apple cider vinegar
*2 tablespoons of green onions (thinly sliced)
*1/2 tablespoon of pumpkin seed oil
*1 teaspoon of brown sugar
*1/2 teaspoon of curry powder
*1/2 teaspoon of garlic powder
*pinch of chili peppers (ground)
*black pepper (ground - to season)

Directions:

Put the shredded cabbage in a serving bowl. In a
separate smaller bowl, mix all the other ingredients
together to form a dressing. Toss the dressing to coat
the cabbage. Refrigerate for at least half an hour before

serving. Store leftovers in the refrigerator.

Cream Corn

Makes 6 servings.

Ingredients:

*6 cups of corn (canned, frozen or husked)
*1 cup of onion (yellow, finely chopped)
*3/4 cup of chicken broth (divided)
*2 tablespoons of olive oil
*1 1/2 tablespoons of lime juice
*1 tablespoon of cilantro (fresh chopped)
*1 tablespoon of Serrano chili pepper (minced)
*salt and pepper to taste

Deseed the Serrano chili pepper before mincing. Add a cup of corn and half of the 3/4 cup of chicken broth to the blender and blend until smooth. Add the 2 tablespoons to a large frying pan and turn heat to medium. Sauté the cup of finely chopped yellow onion with a dash of salt. Pour in the remaining 5 cups of corn and sauté for a couple minutes more to heat through. Add more salt if desired. Pour in the corn and pepper puree mixture and simmer for 2 minutes. Pour in the remaining half of the chicken broth, the 1 1/2 tablespoons of lime juice and the tablespoon of cilantro

and heat through. Add more salt and pepper to season.
Serve immediately.

Mac and Cheese

Makes 6 servings.

Ingredients:

*1 box of macaroni noodles (8oz)
*3/4 cup of liquid non-dairy coffee creamer (make sure it has no whey in it)
*3/4 cup of rice milk
*1 1/2 cups of cheddar cheese substitute
*3 tablespoons of margarine
*3 tablespoons of corn starch
*1 tablespoon of yeast (nutritional)
*1/4 teaspoon of black pepper (ground)
*1/4 teaspoon of paprika
*1/8 teaspoon of mustard powder

Directions:

Cook the macaroni according to the package directions. Drain the water and set aside. In a separate pan melt the 3 tablespoons of margarine and add the 3 tablespoons of corn starch to make a roux over low heat. Mix in the 3/4 cup of non-dairy coffee creamer and the 3/4 cup of rice milk. Whisk to make a white gravy sauce. Stir in the

1 1/2 cups of cheddar cheese substitute until melted and well blended. Stir in the tablespoon of yeast, 1/4 teaspoon of black pepper, 1/4 teaspoon of paprika, and the 1/8 teaspoon of mustard powder. Add the noodles and heat through. Serve hot.

Squash Soup

Makes 4 servings.

Ingredients:

*6 cups of butternut squash (peeled and diced)
*4 slices of bread (cut into bite sized chunks)
*4 cups of chicken broth
*1 cup of onions (chopped)
*1/2 cup of olive oil (divided)
*1 sweet potato (peeled and diced)
*4 garlic cloves (finely chopped)
*2 teaspoons of coriander (ground)
*1/4 teaspoon of salt
*1/4 teaspoon of black pepper (ground)

Directions:

Pour 1/4 cup of olive oil into a large saucepan and turn on medium heat. Sauté the 1 cup of chopped onions and the 3 finely chopped garlic cloves. Stir in the 6 cups of diced butternut squash, diced sweet potato, and the 2 teaspoons of coriander and sauté for 5 minutes. Pour in the 4 cups of chicken broth, turn heat to high, and bring to a boil. Turn the heat down to simmer until squash is soft for about 25 minutes, stirring occasionally. Pour entire contents into a blender or food processor and puree. Pour back into the saucepan and add the 1/4 teaspoon of salt and black pepper. Heat through. Meanwhile take the 4 slices of bread and cut into cubes. Heat 1/4 cup of olive oil in a skillet on medium, add the remaining minced garlic clove and the bread, and toss around while it "fries" for about 7 minutes. Remove from heat and serve with the soup.

Chicken A La King

Makes 4 servings.

Ingredients:

*2 chicken breasts (deboned, skinned)
*8 pearl onions
*1 1/2 cups of chicken broth
*1 cup of ham (cubed)
*1 cup of peas (frozen)
*1 cup of carrot (thinly sliced)
*3 sprigs of parsley
*2 celery leaves (from 2 stalks)
*1 bay leaf
*2 tablespoons of flour (all-purpose)
*2 tablespoons of margarine (melted)
*salt and pepper to taste

Directions:

Add the 2 chicken breasts to a large deep skillet along with the 1 1/2 cups of chicken broth, 3 sprigs of parsley, 2 celery leaves, and the bay leaf. Put a lid on and cook on medium low heat for about 20 minutes. Stir in the 8 pearl onions and the cup of thinly sliced carrots and cook another 10 minutes. Remove the chicken from the skillet and set on a plate to cool. Remove the parsley sprigs, celery leaves and the bay leaf, set aside. Cut the chicken into bite-sized chunks and add into the casserole along with the cups of ham and peas. Take 2 tablespoons of the broth and add to a cup. Whisk in the 2 tablespoons of all-purpose flour along with the melted 2 tablespoons of margarine. Pour the paste back into the broth in the skillet, heat on medium high for 3 minutes, stir constantly to avoid lumps. Pour the broth over the chicken, ham, and peas in the casserole dish.

Heat the casserole dish in the oven for chicken a la king at 400 degrees Fahrenheit for 10 minutes. Serve over rolls or toasted French bread. On the other hand, serve in a cooked piecrust for a chicken pot pie.

Lasagna

Makes 8 servings.

Ingredients:

*16 rice and corn lasagna sheets
*1 3/4 cups of ground beef (cooked)
*1 1/2 cups of rice milk (divided)
*1 zucchini (graded)
*1/2 cup of onion (chopped)
*1/2 cup of carrot (grated)
*2 sprigs of parsley (finely chopped)
*1 garlic clove (finely chopped)
*1 chicken bouillon cube
*1 bay leaf
*2 teaspoons of corn starch
*1 tablespoon of extra virgin olive oil
*1 tablespoon of quinoa grains
*1/4 teaspoon salt (+ more to season)
*3/4 cup of water
*breadcrumbs

Directions:

Brown the ground beef drain and set aside. Add the

tablespoon of olive oil to a skillet and sauté the grated zucchini, 1/2 cups of carrots and onions, chopped garlic clove and the tablespoon of quinoa grains. Stir in the cooked ground beef and the chopped parsley and heat through. Add the 3/4 cup of water with the bouillon cube and stir, cooking over medium heat for 20 minutes. Salt to taste. The mixture will be runny and this is okay. In a separate pan, heat the 1 1/4 cups of rice milk with the bay leaf. Once heated remove from the stove and discard the bay leaf. Add the 2 teaspoons of corn starch to the heated rice milk and heat again, stirring constantly until the sauce thickens. Take off heat as soon as it reaches a thick sauce consistency. Next layer the lasagna by spreading a couple of spoons of meat mixture in the bottom of a 9x13 baking dish, enough to "wet" the bottom. Place a layer of lasagna noodles followed by half of the meat mixture followed by half of the rice milk sauce. Then the last half of the meat sauce, followed by the lasagna noodles, and topped with the white rice milk sauce. Dust the top with breadcrumbs. Cover tightly with foil and cook in a 350 degree Fahrenheit oven for about 35 minutes, until the pasta sheets are al dente. Remove the foil for the last 5 minutes of cook time, then remove pan from oven and allow sitting for 10 minutes before serving.

Cabbage Soup

Makes 4 servings.

Ingredients:

*4 cups of vegetable stock
*2 heads of cabbage (shredded)
*1 tablespoon of soymilk
*white pepper to taste
*salt to taste

Directions:

Place the 2 heads of shredded cabbage in the 4 cups of vegetable stock in a sauce pan and bring to a boil and cook until the cabbage is tender. Salt and pepper to taste. Pour the soup into a food processor or blender and puree. Return to saucepan and add the tablespoon of soymilk, stir and heat through. Serve warm.

"Cheesy" Vegetable Casserole

Makes 8 servings.

Ingredients:

*1 pound of spinach (rinsed and chopped)
*1/2 pound of kale (rinsed and chopped, leaves only)
*1/2 pound of nettles (no thick stems)
*1 box of puff pastry (17.3 oz)
*3 potatoes (sliced and boiled)
*14 oz of mushrooms (white button)
*10 ounces of Monterey Jack cheese substitute
*1 1/4 cups of onion (chopped)
*1 cup of chicken broth
*3 eggs (divided)
*4 tablespoons of coconut oil (divided)
*4 garlic cloves (minced)
*1/8 teaspoon of liquid smoke
*salt and pepper to taste

Directions:

Allow the puff pastry to thaw outside of the package. Takes a little under an hour. Slice the 3 potatoes and boil until tender but not falling apart. Remove from heat and set aside. Heat the 3 tablespoons of coconut oil in a large skillet and add the 1 1/4 cups of onions along with the 4 minced garlic cloves and sauté. Gradually add the pound of chopped spinach, 1/2 pound of chopped kale and 1/2 pound of nettles, slowly stirring, and sautéing. Pour the cup of chicken broth into the greens and continue to cook until the greens are tender. Remove from heat, drain the chicken broth, and set aside. Shred the 10 ounces of imitation Monterey jack cheese and add the 2 eggs, beat slightly and set aside. If the puff pastry is thawed, roll it out and line a 9x9 baking pan, carefully patting down. Mix the cheese and eggs into the greens and place in the refrigerator. Preheat the oven to 350 degrees Fahrenheit. Add 1 tablespoon of coconut oil to a skillet and heat to sauté the 14 oz of white button mushrooms. Sprinkle in the 1/8 teaspoon of liquid smoke and mushrooms are done when they are softened. Add the mushrooms on the puffed pastry in the baking dish, then spoon the greens over the mushrooms, then add the potato slices. Season the potatoes with salt and pepper. Next, carefully place the puffed pastry over the top of the potatoes, carefully sliding the pastry inside the sides of the dish. Beat the third egg and brush the top of the pastry. Carefully set the baking dish on a cookie sheet and bake until the top is golden brown, about 40 minutes. Once done, remove and allow sitting for 10 minutes, then serve while still hot.

Sweet Potato Soup

Makes 8 servings.

Ingredients:

*1 large carton of beef broth (48 oz)
*1 pound of crimini mushrooms (finely chopped)
*5 potatoes (red grated)
*3 stalks of celery (diced)
*2 zucchinis (diced)
*2 leeks (sliced thin)
*1 sweet potato (diced)
*1/2 tablespoon of salt
*1/2 tablespoon of tarragon (dried)
*1/2 tablespoon of parsley (dried)
*1/2 teaspoon of black pepper (ground)

Directions:

Pour the 48 ounces of beef broth in a pot and bring to a boil. Add all the ingredients to the broth stir and simmer with a lid on for 60 minutes or when the vegetables are soft. Serve with bread or crackers.

Chicken and Dumplings

Makes 6 servings.

Ingredients:

*4 chicken breast halves (sliced)
*5 cups of chicken stock
*2 cups of cauliflower
*2 cups of broccoli
*2 cups of green beans
*1 1/3 cup of biscuit mix (make sure it is dairy-free)
*2 eggs
*1/2 teaspoon of corn starch
*water (about 1/3 cup)
*parsley (flat-leaf for garnish)
*salt and pepper to season

Directions:

Rub salt and pepper into the 4 chicken breasts and cook on the grill. Meanwhile pour the 5 cups of chicken stock into a large pot and add the 2 cups of cauliflower, broccoli, green beans and sliced chicken breasts. Bring the mixture to a boil. In a separate bowl add the 2 eggs and beat in the 1/2 teaspoon of corn starch with the 1

1/3 cup of biscuit mix. Add water until it makes a biscuit dough consistency, about 1/3 cup. Spoon the dough into the boiling broth and cook until the dumplings float to the top, for about 8 minutes. Serve immediately.

Turkey Burgers

Makes 4 servings.

Ingredients:

*1 pound of ground turkey
*4 slices of bacon
*4 whole wheat buns
*1/4 cup of onion (finely chopped)
*2 tablespoons of extra virgin olive oil
*2 tablespoons of parsley (flat-leaf chopped)
*4 teaspoons of olive oil mayonnaise
*2 teaspoons of poultry seasoning
*1 teaspoon of basil pesto
*1/2 teaspoon of paprika
*grill seasoning (to taste)
*lettuce
*tomatoes

Directions:

Cook the 4 slices of bacon. In a bowl, add the pound of ground turkey and mix with the 2 teaspoons of poultry seasoning, and 1/2 teaspoon of paprika. Mix in the chopped onions and form into 4 patties. Sprinkle the grill seasoning over each side and cook in a frying pan in the 2 tablespoons of extra virgin olive oil for 5 minutes each side. Meanwhile mix the 4 teaspoons of olive oil mayonnaise with the teaspoon of basil pesto and spread on each side of the bun. Put the cooked turkey patty on the bottom bun and break a slice of bacon in half and put 2 halves on each patty and top with a tomato slice and a lettuce leaf. Enjoy.

Snacks and Desserts

Banana Coconut Honey Oat Bars

Makes 9 servings.

Ingredients:

*1 1/4 cups of oats (regular oat meal)
*1 cup of bananas (mashed)
*1/2 cup of coconut (flakes)
*1/4 cup of flour (all purpose)
*1/4 cup of honey
*1 egg
*2 tablespoons of canola oil
*1 teaspoon of vanilla extract
*1/2 teaspoon of baking soda
*1/4 teaspoon of salt

Directions:

Preheat the oven to 350 degrees Fahrenheit. Spray an 8x8 baking dish with cooking spray. In a bowl, combine the 1 1/4 cups of oats with the 1/4 cup of honey, 2 tablespoons of canola oil and teaspoon of vanilla extract. In a separate bowl, add the 1/4 cup of flour with the 1/2 teaspoon of baking soda and the 1/4 teaspoon of salt and mix. Slightly beat the egg and stir into the oat mixture along with the 1 cup of bananas and 1/2 cup of coconut flakes. Gradually stir in the flour mixture, careful not to over mix. Spread the thick batter into the sprayed 8x8 baking dish and cook until toothpick inserted in the middle comes out clean or about 28 minutes. Cool before serving. Store in the refrigerator.

Pumpkin Pie

Makes 6 to 8 servings.

Ingredients:

*1 pie shell (frozen kind or refrigerator)
*1 can of pumpkin (around 15 oz)
*1 cup of rice milk
*1/2 cup of brown sugar
*2 eggs
*1 1/2 teaspoons of cinnamon (ground)
*1/2 teaspoon of ginger (powdered)
*1/4 teaspoon of nutmeg (ground
*1/4 teaspoon of salt

Directions:

Preheat the oven to 350 degrees Fahrenheit and thaw the pie crust.

Beat the 2 eggs with an electric mixer, until frothy. Gradually add the 1/2 cup of brown sugar, 1 1/2 teaspoons of ground cinnamon, 1/2 teaspoon of powdered ginger, 1/4 teaspoon of salt and 1/4 teaspoon of ground nutmeg. Add the can of pumpkin and the cup of rice milk and beat until blended. Prick holes with a fork on the bottom. Pour the pumpkin batter into the uncooked pie shell. Place pie on a cookie sheet and bake for 45 minutes or until done (when the pumpkin pie filling is no longer runny. Cool before serving.

Cheese Popcorn

Makes 4 servings.

Ingredients:

*1/2 cup of popcorn kernels (unpopped)
*2 tablespoons of olive oil
*2 tablespoons of yeast (nutritional)
*1 tablespoon of margarine
*1 teaspoon of curry powder
*salt to season

Directions:

Het the 2 tablespoons of olive oil in a large pan or stockpot with a lid on medium high heat. Add the 1/2 cup of popcorn kernels and keep the lid on while shaking the pot over the burner until the popping stops. Put popped corn into a large bowl and drizzle melted margarine over it, then sprinkle the 2 tablespoons of nutritional yeast along with the teaspoon of curry powder and salt, toss popcorn to coat and enjoy.

Chocolate Pudding

Makes 4 servings.

Ingredients:

*1 1/2 cups of chocolate rice dream
*2 3/4 tablespoons of cornstarch
*2 1/4 tablespoons of brown sugar (packed)
*1 teaspoon of vanilla extract
*1/8 teaspoon of salt
*1/4 cup of semi-sweet chocolate chips

Directions:

Add the Rice Dream chocolate milk in a mid-sized saucepan along with the 2 3/4 tablespoons of cornstarch, 2 1/4 tablespoons of packed brown sugar, teaspoon of vanilla extract and 1/8 teaspoon of salt. Stir with a whisk or a fork. Turn heat to medium and stir continually as the liquid starts to boil. It will thicken a bit as it boils, turn heat off, and remove. Stir in the 1/4 cup of semi-sweet chocolate chips. Cool a few minutes, then spoon into 4 dessert bowls and serve. Store covered in the refrigerator.

Chocolate Rice Crispy Bars

Makes 12 servings.

Ingredients:

*2 cups of crisp rice cereal
*1 3/4 cups of coconut flakes (divided)
*3/4 cup of semi-sweet chocolate chips
*6 tablespoons of honey
*1/2 teaspoon of vanilla extract

Directions:

Grease an 8x8 baking dish with margarine. In a food processor, add 1 1/2 cups of coconut flakes and chop. Pour in the 6 tablespoons of honey and the 1/2 teaspoon of vanilla extract and blend for another half a minute to mix well. Pour the 2 cups of crisp rice cereal in a large bowl and mix in the remaining 1/4 cup of coconut flakes. Add the coconut, honey paste, and grease your hands with margarine. Then with your fingers incorporate the paste onto the cereal and coconut flakes. Put the sticky mixture into the 8x8 greased pan and press down evenly. Cover with foil and free for 10 to 15 minutes. Meanwhile put the 1/4 cup of semi-sweet chocolate chips into a microwave safe bowl and microwave for 1 minute, stir well. Remove the crisp bars from the freezer and cut into 9 squares. With your hands dip the bar to the half way point on the top of the flat side, then place on a sheet of waxed paper, chocolate side up to cool and dry.

NOTE: Add sugar sprinkles, chopped nuts, or more coconut to the top of the chocolate before it sets if desired.

Coconut Flavored Rice Pudding

Makes 6 servings.

Ingredients:

*2 cups of coconut milk
*2 cups of water
*1/2 cup of sugar (granulated)
*1/2 cup of basmati rice (rinsed)
*1 teaspoon of vanilla extract
*1 teaspoon of cinnamon (ground)

Directions:

In a saucepan, add the 2 cups of water along with the 1/2 cup of granulated sugar and the 1/2 cup of basmati rice. Turn the heat on high and bring the mixture to a boil, stirring occasionally. Once the liquid boils, reduce the heat to simmer and stir often for 20 minutes. Remove from heat and stir in the teaspoon of vanilla extract and teaspoon of ground cinnamon. Spoon into 6 dessert bowls and serve immediately. Store in the refrigerator and serve cold too, if desired.

Crunchy Oatmeal Cookies

Makes two dozen cookies.

Ingredients:

*2 cups of oats
*1 cup of trail mix
*2/3 cup of honey
*1/2 cup of flaxmeal
*4 tablespoons of canola oil
*4 tablespoons of cornstarch
*1teaspoon of vanilla extract
*1 teaspoon of baking powder

Directions:

Preheat the oven to 350 degrees Fahrenheit. Using parchment paper, line a cookie sheet.

Add the 2.3 cup of honey with the 1/2 cup of flaxmeal, 4 tablespoons of canola oil, 4 tablespoons of cornstarch, 1 teaspoon of vanilla extract, and the 1 teaspoon of baking powder. Stir to mix well. Fold in the 2 cups of oats and the 1 cup of trail mix. Grease your hands with margarine and shape into 24 balls and place a dozen at a time on the parchment paper on the cookie sheet. Bake for about 12 minutes, cookies are done when the edges turn golden brown, the top will have a slight sheen. Allow to cool before serving.

Yellow Cake

Makes 8 servings.

Ingredients:

*1 1/2 cups of flour (all-purpose)
*1 cup of soy milk
*1/2 cup of canola oil
*1 cup of sugar (granulated)
*1 tablespoon of vanilla extract
*1 tablespoon of vinegar
*1 teaspoon of baking soda
*1/2 teaspoon of salt

Preheat oven to 350 degrees Fahrenheit. Spray an 8 inch cake pan with cooking spray with oil and flour. In a bowl add the 1 1/2 cups of all-purpose flour along with the 1 cup of granulated sugar, teaspoon of baking soda and 1/2 teaspoon of salt. Stir to mix. Pour in the 1 cup of soy milk, 1/2 cup of canola oil, and the tablespoon of vanilla extract, using a whisk to blend into a smooth and creamy batter. Stir in the tablespoon of vinegar quickly and immediately pour into the prepared cake pan. Bake until a toothpick inserted in the middle comes out clean, about 30 minutes. Cool on a wire rack before removing from pan, serve, or frost and serve.

Fudge

Makes about 24 servings.

Ingredients:

*4 cups of confectioners' sugar
*1/2 cup of almond milk
*1/2 cup of cocoa powder (unsweetened)
*1/2 cup of semi-sweet chocolate chips
*2 tablespoons of margarine
*1 teaspoon of vanilla extract

Directions:

Mix together the 4 cups of confectioners' sugar with the 1/2 cup of cocoa powder. Add the 1/2 cup of semi-sweet chocolate chips. Pour the 1/2 cup of almond milk into a saucepan and turn heat to medium high, stirring constantly with a whisk. When the milk boils, turn heat off, remove saucepan from burner, and pour immediately into the sugar and cocoa mixture. Stir until all the chocolate chips melt. Grease an 8x8 pan with margarine and pour the fudge into the pan. Cover and refrigerate for a couple of hours. Cut into 24 squares.

Apple Crumb Dessert

Makes 6 servings.

Ingredients:

*6 apples
*1 1/2 cups of flour (self-rising)
*1/2 cup of almonds (sliced)
*1/2 cup of brown sugar
*1/2 cup of margarine
*1/2 cup of water
*1/4 cup of sugar (granulated)
*1 1/2 teaspoons of cinnamon

Directions:

Preheat the oven to 375 degrees Fahrenheit. Prepare the 6 apples by peeling and coring, then slice thin. Lay the apple slices in a pie pan and sprinkle with the 1/4 cup of granulated sugar and the 1 1/2 teaspoons of cinnamon. Pour the 1/2 cup of water over the top. In a bowl, add the 1 1/2 cups of self-rising flour with the 1/2 cup of almonds and 1/2 cup of brown sugar and mix. Stir in the 1/2 cup of margarine until it turns into "crumbs". Sprinkle the crumbs over the apples. Place on a cookie sheet in the oven and bake until the crumbs turn a golden brown about half an hour.

Dairy Free Diet Conclusion

Any diet plan needs the direction of your healthcare provider. While all of these recipes are dairy-free make sure to read the ingredients of the foods you use to make these recipes to be one hundred percent certain they are milk free. Always go over your diet plan with your healthcare provider, especially if you are eating dairy free for health reasons. These recipes should provide weeks worth of meals and snacks while avoiding dairy foods altogether.